"... a fast-paced thriller with a suspenseful ending."

—*The Sunday Oklahoman*

"*NO DEADLY DRUG* ... fascinates and educates. Although a work of fiction, much of it is based on events that have or could have taken place."

—Jere E. Goyan, Dean, School of Pharmacy, University of California, San Francisco, former head of the Food and Drug Administration

"A finely drawn portrait of a crusading media doc at war with a big, Machiavellian drug company. Hero Gabe Austin is as real and believable as tomorrow's sound bite. A SUPERB MEDICAL THRILLER!"

—Dean Ornish, M.D., author of
Dr. Dean Ornish's Guide to Reversing Heart Disease

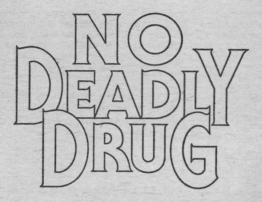

NO DEADLY DRUG

TOM FERGUSON and JOE GRAEDON

POCKET BOOKS

New York   London   Toronto   Sydney   Tokyo   Singapore

This book is a work of fiction. Names, characters, places, and incidents are either products of the author's imagination or are used fictitiously. Any resemblance to actual events or locales or persons, living or dead, is entirely coincidental.

POCKET BOOKS, a division of Simon & Schuster Inc.
1230 Avenue of the Americas, New York, NY 10020

Copyright © 1992 by Tom Ferguson

ISBN: 0-671-74870-X

First Pocket Books paperback printing December 1993

10 9 8 7 6 5 4 3 2 1

POCKET and colophon are registered trademarks of Simon & Schuster Inc.

Cover art by Don Brautigam

Printed in the U.S.A.

*This book is for Meredith and Adrienne,
who believed in it from the beginning,
for Terry, who made it all possible,
and in memory of Sid Graedon,
who gave us inspiration
and who never knew a book he didn't love.*

I swear by Apollo the Physician
that I will practice medicine to the best of my ability
and solely for the benefit of my patients.
I will abstain from all manner of mischief and corruption
and I will prescribe no deadly drug. . . .

—Hippocratic Oath

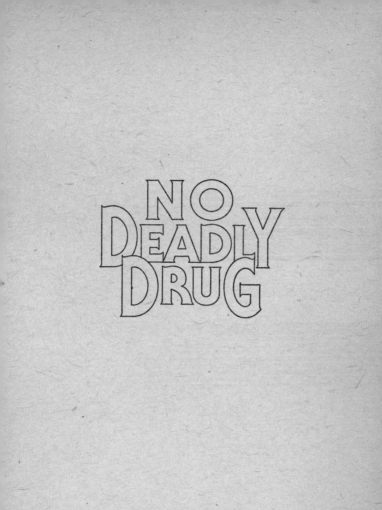

1

Gabe Austin leaned back against the battered wall of the hospital elevator, his scrubs clammy against the cold metal. The emergency room had been a zoo from the moment he'd started his shift. He'd been working without a break for nearly forty-eight hours. He would begin to hear the voices soon. He could almost hear them now, faint overtones through the deep throbbing of the elevator motor, many floors below.

It was something he never thought of in his more rested moments, the dim, sweet voices that spoke to him in the hiss of the oxygen line, the steady purr of the respirator. He sometimes imagined that they were the voices of his patients who had died. They had frightened him once. Now he found them strangely comforting.

Gabe was an inch over six feet. His face was all flat planes and sharp angles. At age 34 he still weighed the same—178 pounds—as fourteen years earlier, when he had set the Cal–Berkeley school record for kicking nineteen field goals in a row. He got off on the sixth floor, receiving the serene nods of two nursing sisters returning from Mass.

His shaggy hair and his stained, rumpled blue scrub

suit stood out among the three-piece suits of the attendings, the bright white jackets of the medical residents, and the crisp green scrubs of the two surgical teams. They were all helping themselves to coffee and doughnuts provided by the drug company of the day. Gabe found their early morning heartiness vaguely distasteful.

". . . The surgeons want to explore her but the damn OR schedule is completely full."

". . . They want you to file another goddamn incident report every time some old gomer falls out of bed."

". . . Started losing weight again, so we started her on hyperal pumped into the subclavian . . ."

". . . Three previous admissions for pancreatic CA, with two exploratories and a course of chemo at General . . ."

A fresh-faced young woman he did not know, obviously the drug company sales rep, stood behind a long table of plastic giveaways and brightly colored promotional literature. None of the doctors paid her the least attention.

A friend from the B team punched him lightly on the arm. "Hey, Gabe, baby. How are things down in the pit?"

"Hey, Carter. Just dandy. Excuse me. I'm still working."

He pushed his way toward the gleaming coffee urn, poured a cup, and drank it, postponing the confrontation that was to come. He closed his eyes and felt his center of consciousness rise from his pelvic basin, past his liver and spleen, and into his chest. It paused for a few seconds at his throat. As he leaned down to refill his cup, he felt it reach the pulsing darkness behind his eyes.

Gabe made his way down the long sixth-floor hallway to the doctors' lounge, stopping to check his reflection in the dark glass of an office door. He was painfully aware of the disreputable state of his scrub suit, the prominent beating of his heart. He reached up under his shirt, placing his fingertips just below his left nipple, closing his eyes to feel the contours of his first and second heart sounds.

Just garden-variety anxiety tachycardia, he assured himself. For a fleeting moment he wished he hadn't asked Kate to meet him at the hospital. He had been so surprised and pleased when she had finally called, months after he had received her letter, that he had chosen the earliest possible time. She had always had a knack for catching him at his worst. He took a deep breath, bit his lip, and, holding the white Styrofoam cup before him, made his way into the leathery darkness of the doctors' lounge.

At first he thought no one was there. Then he was aware of movement in the library alcove at the back of the room. His face grew hot and he was again shaken by the rapid beating of his heart.

It was Kate all right, her round, Irish face, her expressive mouth, her deep, intelligent eyes. He was struck by the change in her appearance. He remembered her as a pretty, dark-eyed girl in long hair and jeans, her body cloaked in an ample layer of baby fat. She was older now. The extra pounds had dropped away. Her skin was drawn tight against her cheekbones, her dark hair cut short and curled. She wore a well-tailored gray suit with an elegant white lace blouse. She looked fit and happy, full of energy and enthusiasm.

He had a fleeting vision of her hurt, angry, tear-stained face, telling him she never wanted to see him again. They'd been walking across the wet fields that surrounded the Yale Bowl. It had been raining and the wind had whipped her long, rain-soaked hair across her face as she accused him of being so wrapped up in medicine that he had no time in his life for her.

"Kate?" he said softly.

"Well I'll be damned. There he is. Still alive." She twisted her lower jaw to one side, raising her eyebrows. "A few touches of gray, but still wearing the same goddamn scrub suit." She had a sure, quiet intensity that was new to him. Gabe was surprised to see that there were tears in her eyes. He had been expecting recriminations.

"Welcome to San Francisco," he said.

"Yeah. Shit. It only took me ten years to get here." She hesitated, watching him closely, her arms crossed on her chest. "So how are you, Gabe?"

"Surviving," he said. "A little tired right now."

"You want to put that coffee down and come give me a hug or what?"

Then she was in his arms, squeezing him around the ribs. He was acutely aware of her body against him. She smelled of shampoo and sleep and green apples.

She nuzzled at his shoulder. "Oh, God," she said, "it's *so* good to see you. Does . . . does it feel any different?"

"No." He shook his head. "The left one?"

She nodded. "You don't know what it meant to me, to have you talk to my doctors like you did."

"Happy to do it," he said. "Your tests all been good?"

She nodded and smiled, holding up crossed fingers. "So far. You scared my poor surgeon to death."

"I didn't want him to lose his concentration."

"He didn't. The operation was a complete success. How's your dad, by the way?" Kate had met Gabe's father years ago in New Haven. They had taken a special liking to each other.

"He's fine," Gabe said. "He got married again a couple of years ago. He and my stepmother have a real estate office in Santa Rosa. His memory's not what it once was, but they're doing great. Your parents okay?"

She held up crossed fingers again. "So far, so good, thank God."

"And Russell?"

"Russell and I split up. Almost a year ago," Kate said.

"Whose idea was that?"

"Mine, mostly. I'd decided to call it quits before they found the lump." Gabe could feel the blood pounding in his chest. Perhaps she had decided to come back to him after all.

She locked her hands behind his waist, leaned back, and looked up at him. "I have a great job up in Marin. Running a big corporate wellness program. They give me plenty of time to train and it pays more money than I ever dreamed of."

"How long have you been here?"

"Just over three months."

"Why did you wait so long to call?"

"I . . . I had my reasons." She reached up to brush a lock of hair from his face. "You never told me why you left UC," she said. "I heard they'd given you tenure."

"They did. I gave it up when they asked me to resign."

"Why?"

"I reported one of my colleagues to the local DA's office."

"For what?"

"Wrongful death."

She smiled. "They must have loved that."

"My chairman felt it was inappropriate."

"So we've both had a change," she said.

He nodded. "I've been following your career in the sports pages," he said. "I want to hear all about it." He recalled their lovemaking, years ago. She had been a marathoner of sorts even then.

"At breakfast." She tugged at his hand. "Go change your clothes. I'm starving."

"We've got to go back downstairs," he said. A familiar feeling of uneasiness crept up on him. "I have one last patient coming in."

Kate looked up at the ceiling and rolled her eyes. "Back to reality," she said. "One thing you can count on with Gabe Austin—he will *always* have one last patient coming in."

"It's not typical, dammit. She's almost family."

"Almost?" Kate raised her eyebrows.

"She's Julia's niece," he said uneasily. "Her name's Lindsey."

A flicker of discomfort passed across Kate's eyes. She frowned. "Julia's the woman from UC you were living with for a while? The physician's assistant?"

"Uh-huh. Lindsey used to stay with us a lot when she was just a kid. Her mother called me this morning. They're coming in by ambulance. I promised I'd see her."

They jammed into a corner of the elevator to accommodate an old Vietnamese man on crutches, accompanied by what appeared to be his extended family. When they got out on the first floor, the security guard looked up from his desk in surprise.

"You back already, Doc? I thought you finally got out of this nuthouse."

"Just crazy in the head, Albert. You know where Robbie is?"

"Back in the radio room. The big boss's looking for you too. There he is now."

A nervous, balding man of about sixty came hurrying purposefully around the corner. He wore a crisp, well-tailored blue suit and carried an unlit pipe the way a Greek might carry a set of worry beads. A few sparse hairs stood above the liver spots on his scalp like so many twitching antennae.

"Austin. There you are. I need to talk to you." He pointed the stem of his pipe at the bloodstains on Gabe's trousers. "Why don't you put on a clean set of scrubs, for Christ's sake?"

"Relax, Sid. I'm just about out of here. This is Kate Reiley. Sid Crowell, chief of medicine."

"Oh, yes. Dr. Reiley. The . . . ah . . . the marathon runner." Crowell sneaked a quick glance at her chest. Kate gave Gabe a pained look.

"What is it you wanted, Sid?" Gabe said. "I've got a patient coming in."

Crowell frowned again, clearing his throat. "I understand you've had one of our liver cases down here all night," he said. "A chronic GI bleeder at that."

"Sammy Denton? He's not bleeding. I'm just giving him some IV vitamins." He turned to Kate. "Sammy's this sweet little homeless guy who makes speeches about Trotsky in the McDonald's parking lot."

Crowell tapped the bowl of his pipe against the palm of his left hand. "He's been in and out of here a dozen times, Austin. Always when *you're* on duty. He's never been admitted and he's never had a liver biopsy. Now in my book that's bad—"

"He's barely got any liver tissue *left*. You let those goons of yours loose on him, he's going to be checking into that big liver ward in the sky."

"Excuse me, gentlemen," Albert stepped forward

and put a hand on Gabe's arm. "Dr. Dugan says she needs Dr. Austin right now."

Crowell glowered. "We'll talk about this later."

"Sure thing, Sid. How about the next meeting of the human experimentation review committee?"

Crowell flushed. "Damn you, Austin. That's Jackson's bunch. He'd do anything he could . . ."

Gabe backed away holding up both his hands. "Sorry, Sid. Duty calls."

He led Kate down the hallway, past a frail elderly man sleeping on a wheeled stretcher. A slow-moving janitor was mopping up a puddle under a water fountain.

"Wow," Kate said, hurrying along beside him. "You guys really get into it. Isn't he your boss?"

"Don't remind me." Gabe shook his head in disgust. "Sid needs a lot of liver biopsies for a study he's doing. He's actually a pretty good researcher, but whoever decided to make him chief of medicine should be strung up by the spleen."

He waved her into a glass-walled room where a tall, graceful young woman in a scrub suit and headphones was leaning against a high counter, speaking into a microphone.

"What's that?" she was saying. "Uh-huh. Well why *can't* you get a blood pressure? And her heart sounds? Uh-huh. And the pulse? Well why doesn't she have a blood pressure then? Yes, I wish you *would* try again. I'll hold on."

She turned to them, pushing back her hair in exasperation. "It's Lindsey Troutman," she said. "The mother called one of those tiny ambulance companies with no on-board monitoring equipment. You wonder where they get these . . ." She frowned suddenly and turned back to the microphone. "You *still* can't get

8

a blood pressure? Well what does her skin look like? Is she cold and pale or warm and flushed?''

Gabe put a hand on her shoulder and made a flipping motion. Robbie nodded and turned a knob on the counter. A nervous, defensive young man's voice came over the ceiling speaker.

"She seems real hot to me, ma'am. And she's real red in the face." The siren in the background made his voice difficult to hear.

"And her heart sounds are okay?"

"Yes, ma'am. As far as I can tell. Her pulse is real fast."

"All right. Hold on a minute." She put a hand on Gabe's arm. "They're coming in from Bernal Heights. The mother found the girl on the kitchen floor, screaming and holding her head. Sounds like she's in shock."

Gabe picked up the microphone. "The headache is her chief complaint, is it?" he said.

"That's what the mother says."

"What are her vital signs?" Gabe said.

"The pulse is 120 and pounding. She's got extrasystoles all over the place. Respiration's about 30. The temperature is 101.2. I haven't been able to get a blood pressure sir. It must be pretty low. She's really thrashing around."

"Is she conscious, confused, delirious, or what?"

"I'd have to say delirious, sir."

"Does she have a stiff neck?"

"She wouldn't hardly let me touch her head, sir. I'd guess she probably does."

"Pupils equal and reactive?"

"Far as I can tell. Hard to see with her thrashing around like that."

"She taken any drugs?"

"Hold on, sir. I'll ask the mother." They could

hear the siren and the sound of car horns. *"No sir. No drugs that she knows of."*

"So what's your impression?"

"Me?" There was a moment's silence. *"I really couldn't say, sir. I just hope to God I never have a headache like the one this kid's got."*

"All right," Gabe said. "Put in an IV of D_5W at maximum flow. Keep trying to get a pressure. And tell Mrs. Troutman that Dr. Austin and Dr. Dugan will be waiting at the hospital."

2

There was no place in the ER to talk privately, so Gabe and Kate went out through the automatic glass doors to the ambulance unloading area. The city was still nearly dark. The park across the street was wrapped in a dim, moist haze. There were rainbows around the streetlights.

Gabe had not been outside—nor had he been to sleep—for forty-eight hours. He leaned back against the high metal railing and looked up at the thick concrete canopy protecting them from the drizzle. Kate paced back and forth, her trench coat blowing against her body, her arms folded against the damp breeze that carried the smell of the ocean. They could hear the siren now, coming up Fell Street, still several blocks away.

"Lindsey is a very special kid," Gabe said. "Getting to know her has been one of the nicer things that's happened to me."

"How old is she?" Kate asked.

"Seventeen. She's a senior at Lincoln High, my alma mater. A hell of an actress. She calls me Uncle Gabe."

"So her mom is Julia's sister?" Kate said.

"Yeah. Her dad's a pediatrician at San Francisco General. He's away at a medical meeting. Lindsey and I always hit it off, even when she was just a kid. A year ago she called me, pregnant and terrified. I ended up taking her in for an abortion. She didn't want her parents to know."

"Well, obviously you need to see her." Kate stood looking out at the rain. "I guess I had some fantasy of a long, romantic breakfast. But if she needs you, she needs you." She squeezed his hand. "I don't know why I'm being such a dope. What can I do to help?"

"Come in and lend a hand. We're short staffed."

"I'm a little rusty at hospital medicine, but I'll do whatever I can." Kate punched him lightly on the shoulder, then leaned back against his chest. "Just don't forget about breakfast," she said.

They stood looking at the red lights flashing through the trees in the park across the street. The siren sank to a dying whine. The ambulance, high, white, and square, swung around the corner and bumped up over the sidewalk. The driver and the attendant opened the back doors, pulled out the stretcher, popped down the wheels, and headed for the sliding glass doors at a run, pushing the stretcher ahead of them. A short, plump woman got out of the ambulance and hurried after them.

Lindsey's slight body was bound to the stretcher by wide gray straps across her chest and knees. She wore a red plaid bathrobe over white pajamas. She writhed against the straps, gasping for breath, twisting her head from side to side and shielding her eyes with her right hand. Her blond hair was tangled and matted with sweat. All poise, all control, was gone. This was no bright, eager, intelligent young actress. This was a miserable, suffering child.

"She looks awful," Kate whispered.

The plump woman came up from behind and clung to Gabe's arm. She wore a white peasant blouse with embroidery around the neck. The bright embroidery thread had left a faint stain on the white fabric. She had been crying and her thick glasses had slipped down on her nose.

"Oh, Gabe. Thank God you're here." She held on to him the way a castaway might clutch a life preserver. "What's wrong with my baby?"

Gabe put an arm around her shoulders and led her in through the automatic glass doors. Kate followed closely behind them. "Margaret," he said. "Tell me what happened."

Lindsey's mother shook her head helplessly. "She got up early to videotape an assignment for her acting class. A little later she came upstairs for an aspirin. She said her head hurt and things looked funny. Then I heard her screaming. When I went downstairs she was lying on the kitchen floor."

The ambulance attendants were waiting with the stretcher inside. "Where do you want her, Doc?"

"Put her in number three," Gabe said. He turned to Margaret. "Anything wrong with her last night?"

12

"No. She was fine." She took off her glasses and wiped her eyes with the back of her hand.

"I need to take a look at her now," Gabe said, prying her hands away. "Annie's going to take you back to the family waiting room. You going to be okay?"

"Oh, don't worry about *me*. Take care of my little girl."

The two ambulance attendants had wheeled the stretcher into cubicle 3.

Gabe stood between them. Together the three men slipped their arms under the girl's body and transferred her to the examining table. Lindsey felt light and hot in his arms. Her muscles quivered and her head needed support. It was not a good sign.

It was eight-fifteen and the nurses from the morning shift were full of energy. Lucille, a stolid vocational nurse from the neighborhood, and Elsa, the quiet, competent young team leader, got Lindsey out of her pajamas and into a white hospital gown. The girl twisted and writhed, rolling her head from side to side, as though battling some invisible demon.

"Dr. Austin? She's really thrashing around. Any chance we could sedate her?" Betty, a recent nursing-school graduate, was a heavy girl with a puffy face and bleached blond hair. She was having trouble getting the blood pressure cuff around Lindsey's arm.

Gabe shook his head. "Not before we figure out what's going on." He introduced Kate to the nurses and asked her to help Betty.

"Pleased to meet you, Doctor," Betty said. "If you could just hold her arm out so I can get this cuff on . . . Yes. Like that. Great."

Gabe put his hand on Lindsey's forehead. It felt hot. He pressed two fingers to the side of her neck. Her pulse was fast and strong. When he put a hand behind her head and tried to bring her chin down to touch her chest, she screamed and tore at his hands with her fingernails.

Robbie stepped in and pulled the curtain closed behind her. "So what do you think?" she asked.

"Looks like we've got a stiff neck, headache, and fever in a seventeen-year-old girl." He turned to Kate. She was holding Lindsey's left arm straight out from her body while Betty pumped up the blood pressure cuff. "Even a wellness doc should be able to diagnose this one."

"Meningitis?"

"That's what it looks like." He put a hand on Elsa's shoulder. "We'll need a spinal tap."

The young team leader nodded, writing on her clipboard order sheet. "You'll need the mother's permission. She'll want to talk to you anyway."

"Doctor," Betty said. "I'm not getting a blood pressure."

"No?"

Betty shook her head, upset with herself. "No. I'm sorry. Nothing."

Gabe took the girl's radial and femoral pulses on each side, feeling the usual mild embarrassment as he palpated the cleft between her pelvis and her upper leg. Lindsey's pulse was strong—too strong. It felt like a tiny hammer tapping against his finger.

"Funny, the ambulance guy couldn't get it either," Gabe said. "She's got a good strong pulse. Try the other arm. It may be low, but there's got to be *something*."

Betty bit her lower lip. She and Kate moved to the other side of the table and began wrapping the cuff around Lindsey's right arm.

"Robbie, after I get the tap, would you do a set of blood cultures? If she's got meningitis it may have gotten into her circulation."

"Sure thing, Gabe." She seemed pleased to have been given something to do.

Gabe picked up an ophthalmoscope, pulled back Lindsey's left eyelid, and tried to look in through the pupil. The girl's eyelashes began to flutter. She tried to pull away.

"Lindsey. Can you hear me?" Gabe tried to bend her neck forward again but she screamed and began to hyperventilate.

Wait a minute, he told himself. *There's something wrong here. There's no way this girl can be in shock.* He took the penlight from his pocket and pulled back one eyelid, but she clawed at his wrist and turned her head away.

"Lindsey. Hold still, dammit," Gabe said. "It's okay. You're at the hospital."

"What? . . . The hospital?" Her eyelids fluttered again. After a minute she opened her eyes.

"Oh, Uncle Gabe. My God. It hurts . . . It hurts . . ."

"When did it start hurting?"

". . . so bad . . . Oh, God, Uncle Gabe, make it stop."

"I'm still not getting a blood pressure, Doctor."

"For Christ's sake, Betty! Do I have to come take it myself? She's lying here talking to me and you're telling me she's got no blood pressure? Elsa, you try it, will you?"

Elsa rested a hand on the younger nurse's shoulder as she took over the cuff.

"Oh, God . . . Somebody . . . Oh pleeease. Do something to make it stop. *Pleeeeeeease!*"

Lindsey's whole body began to tremble. Tears spilled down her cheeks. It seemed to Gabe as if she were looking up at him from beneath many fathoms of water. He asked her another question, but she was twisting from side to side, moaning and sobbing, and did not respond.

3

Here's the permission form. Have Annie take it out to her mother," Gabe said to a nurse's aide stepping back into the cubicle. "We all set for the tap?"

"All ready, Doctor."

Lucille had positioned Lindsey on her left side, her bare back toward the door. She held one powerful arm behind the girl's neck, the other behind her knees. Lindsey lay curled in a ball, her forehead and kneecaps nearly touching, the pale ridge of her spine bowed out over the side of the table.

"Doctor," Elsa said. "I have a pressure. It's 244 over 208."

"*What?* Are you kidding?" Normal pressure for a girl Lindsey's age and weight was about 100 over 65.

Elsa shook her head. "It's 244 over 208," she repeated. "I checked it twice. Would you like to try it yourself?"

Gabe shook his head. "No. Christ. She's in hypertensive crisis." No one had pumped up the cuff high enough, which made it easy to miss an abnormally high pressure.

"Good work, Elsa," Gabe said. "We're going to need a new pressure every five minutes. Kate, will you do that?"

Kate nodded. "Sure. Blood pressures I can handle." She took over the cuff. Gabe was relieved to see that she now seemed totally involved with the effort to do what they could for the girl.

"Call it out every time you get a new one. And write them down, will you—along with the time. Let's get that tap. Then we'll start working on her pressure. Who's on call for neuro?"

Elsa put a pad and pen on the counter behind Kate. "Lew Watkins," she said.

"Thank God. Have Annie call and get him in here—stat. Betty, I want a number 12 intercath and a bottle of Ringer's. After I finish the tap we'll get some bloods—two red tops, one lavender, one green. We'll take an extra red top, too, just in case. Put her name on it and tape it to the back of the supply cabinet." He caught Kate's eye. Taking an extra blood tube was a trick he'd picked up on a medical clerkship they'd done together. If another blood test was needed later, they'd already have a specimen.

"Have Annie call the EKG tech, stat. Come on, people. Let's *move*. Jesus, no wonder she has a headache. She could stroke out on us if we don't get that pressure down."

Gabe palpated the ridge of the girl's spine, locating the space between her fourth and fifth lumbar vertebrae. He wiped the area with Betadine, scrubbed his hands at the sink, pulled on a pair of sterile gloves, and injected the local anesthetic.

Lindsey gasped as the spinal needle went into her back, but Lucille, talking to her in a low, soothing voice, was able to keep her still. Gabe held the long needle in place with his gloved hand and detached the syringe. If the spinal fluid was cloudy, it could indicate meningitis. A drop of fluid seeped out, hovered on the lip of the needle socket, then dripped onto the gray tile floor.

"Looks clear enough," Gabe said. He attached the plastic pressure gauge and watched the spinal fluid rise inside it, reflecting the pressure inside the spinal canal. It was only slightly above normal, about what you'd expect with her elevated blood pressure. He removed the gauge and held a sterile bottle under the needle socket so the spinal fluid could drip into it. He collected another sample in a test tube. He then withdrew the needle, cleaned and bandaged the puncture site, and sent Betty to the microbiology lab with the sterile specimen. He took the test tube into the tiny ER laboratory, spread a sample on a microscope slide, fixed it in the flame of a Bunsen burner, stained it, and put it under the microscope. There were no bacteria to be seen.

"Robbie, you can forget those blood cultures," he said, stepping back into the cubicle. "The spinal fluid looks normal. No blood in it, either, thank God." Blood in the spinal fluid could indicate a stroke. "We need that EKG. Betty, put a three-way on that IV setup, will you? Lucille, get me a cath urine for a complete urinalysis with culture and sensitivity."

Gabe went to the head of the table and began working his fingers over the girl's skull, searching for evidence of a blow to the head. Her hair was thick and glossy. There was no sign of an injury.

A middle-aged Asian woman in a surgical cap rolled a compact white machine into the cubicle. Gabe watched as she applied the shiny EKG gel, then connected a series of small suction cups to Lindsey's chest. She made sure the leads were properly positioned, then ran off a long paper strip on the machine.

"The IV's all set up for you, Doctor," Betty said.

"Good. When it's in I'll want 5 cc's of Hyperstat. Kate, how are you at reading EKGs?"

"So-so."

"Have a look at this one after you take your next reading." He found a deep vein on the inside of Lindsey's arm, scrubbed again, and put on a fresh pair of gloves. Betty broke open the sterile tray with the catheter and the tubing.

"Her pressure's 248 over 210," Kate said. "Still going up."

Gabe took a deep breath, let half of it out, pushed the sharp point of the intercath needle through the skin, and threaded it up into the vein. He withdrew the solid metal core and attached a length of plastic tubing to the catheter, letting the blood run up into the clear tube. Betty taped the assembly to Lindsey's arm and began filling the blood tubes.

"Dr. Austin?" Elsa held out a small syringe. "Here's the Hyperstat you wanted—5 cc's."

"Go ahead and push it in."

"Gabe," Kate said. "You might want to come look at this." She was peering down at the EKG slip. "She's got a mild arrhythmia with a small ST segment depression."

Gabe nodded. "That'd be from her high blood pressure. If we don't get it down it's going to damage her heart."

Lindsey was lying still now, her head back, mouth open, breathing in quick, shallow gasps. Gabe picked up the ophthalmoscope and examined the retina of her right eye. The optic disk was pale against the deep red of the retinal field, like a full moon at sunset. The tiny arteries in her retinas looked normal. There was none of the bulging of the disk that would indicate increased pressure inside her skull.

As suddenly and unmistakably as a circuit breaker

tripping, a warning sounded somewhere in the back of Gabe's brain: Jennifer Cross. Jennifer Cross was a twenty-three-year-old woman who'd died of a blood clot in her brain. She'd been a heavy smoker and had used birth control pills. Her family had sued the drug company and had received a settlement of three-quarters of a million dollars.

"Somebody go ask her mother if Lindsey smokes," he said. "And see if she's on the Pill."

Lindsey's left retina had a medium-sized bleeder just above the optic nerve. There was another near the macula. That would explain the problem with her vision. Gabe turned away from the examining table. Kate was looking up from the blood pressure cuff.

"Pressure's 250 over 212," she said. "It's bad, isn't it?"

Gabe nodded. "Bad enough," he said. If she was blowing vessels in her retina she could be blowing them in her brain as well.

"Doctor. She's trying to sit up."

Lindsey was up on one elbow. Her eyes were open but unfocused. Her lips were moving but she made no sound. Gabe put a hand on her shoulder.

"Lindsey. Can you hear me?"

"Oh, God," she said, her face suddenly pale. "Uncle Gabe? Is that you?"

"Yeah, it's me. I'm here, kiddo."

"What's wrong? What's happening?"

"We're not sure yet. Your blood pressure is real high. Just lie back down."

"I . . . I think I'm going to . . ."

"Betty. Puke basin. Quick." As Betty bent down to open a door in the side cabinet, Lindsey leaned over the side of the table and vomited a large quantity of bright green fluid onto the back of her uniform trousers. Betty gasped, tried to stand up, bumped her head on the marble counter, and sat down hard on the floor. Elsa stepped around her, got the basin, and helped Lindsey lean forward so that most of her second effort went into it.

Lew Watkins stepped in through the green curtains. "Hey there, Gabe," he said. "This Alex's daughter, is it?" He was a pale, immensely competent little man with a heavy jaw, thin, graying hair, and clear brown eyes. He wore a blue rain parka and soft, golden corduroys and looked like a kindly, fiftyish minister who had wandered into L. L. Bean.

"Lew. Great. Am I glad to see *you*."

Lew bent over the table. "Hello, Lindsey. I'm Dr. Watkins. Can you hear me?"

There was no answer. She writhed back and forth on the table, her head back, her hair trailing down over the side. Watkins felt her pulse, then asked Betty to help him hold her head still while he lifted both eyelids and looked at the pupils.

"Tell me about her," he said.

Gabe told him. "I sent bloods and gave her 5 cc's of Hyperstat. No response to it yet."

A curly blond head appeared between the curtains. "Positive for the Pill. And she does smoke."

"Gabe. Come here a second." Lew put a hand on Gabe's arm and led him to an empty cubicle down the hall. "You've just finished a forty-eight-hour shift, right?"

"Yeah. So?"

"So you're obviously exhausted, my friend. For goodness' sake, why don't you let somebody else—"

"I can't, Lew. She's a friend. I promised her mom I'd take care of her."

"Tell you what," Watkins said. "I'll take her on as my own private patient, so that you can go home."

"Jesus, Lew. I appreciate it. I really do. But you're on call. You could be . . ."

"Gabe?" Kate's voice was tinged with alarm. "Her pressure's still going up. It's 255 over 215."

The two men looked at each other. "Another 5 of Hyperstat?" Gabe asked.

Watkins nodded. "Better make it 10," he said.

Gabe gave Elsa the order. Watkins bent over the girl, the ophthalmoscope in his hand. "Bleeders on both sides now. It doesn't look good," he said. "You're sure she's not taking Marplan or Nardil or anything like that?" These were monoamine oxidase inhibitors, drugs that could produce a hypertensive crisis.

"Not that we know of."

Watkins shook his head. "The question is, has she had a cerebral incident that's causing the hypertension, or is it the hypertension that's causing the bleeding? I'm beginning to think we may need a CT scan."

Kate took the stethoscope out of her ears, watching their faces. "Her pressure is 260 over 218," she said.

"Damn," Watkins said. "Still not responding. And it's already affecting her heart. We'd better get her into an ice pack." He turned to Elsa. "Can we get a couple of cubic feet of ice?"

She nodded. "I'll get an orderly to bring some down from the cafeteria."

"I don't like it, Lew," Gabe said. "With smoking and the Pill, I can't help thinking it's got to be a clot. You think we should thin her out a little?"

"Heparin, you mean?" Watkins squeezed his chin between thumb and forefinger. "Not till we get the bloods back. She *could* be bleeding into her brain. If she is and we thin her out, you can just about kiss her goodbye."

Gabe nodded. If she was already bleeding, the heparin could make it worse. A dark wave of remorse swept over him. He should have thought of that. *Too damn tired,* he told himself. The voices floated on the edge of his hearing. They were growing louder, calling him away. He was glad Lew was there.

"Until we know for sure what's happening in her brain, all we can do is keep treating her arteries," Watkins said. "I'm surprised we haven't budged her pressure yet. That's not good. Not good at all."

Annie's head appeared again between the curtains. "Hematology just called. Here's your white count." She handed Gabe a small yellow sheet of paper.

"It's 7.4 with a normal differential," Gabe said. "So much for meningitis."

"I hate to say it, but this just could be another Jennifer Cross," Watkins said. "The pieces don't quite fit," he began, "but then again—"

"You think a CT scan would tell us?"

"It might."

"The pressure is 266 over 220," Kate said.

"Damn. Still going up," Gabe said.

"She's not responding to the Hyperstat," Lew said. "I don't like this at all."

An orderly hurried in, a heavy red plastic bucket of ice in each hand.

"I don't think we can wait any longer," Lew said. "Let's set up that ice pack on a gurney. We need that scan right now."

Gabe stepped out through the curtains. "Annie, call the CT unit. Tell them Lindsey needs a scan, stat, and we're on our way."

4

A young black man wearing a short white jacket and a single gold earring was waiting for them at the door of the CT scanner suite. His name tag read JIMMY FIRBANK, RADIOLOGY TECHNICIAN. He took Lindsey's stretcher and rolled it toward the gleaming white scanner.

Gabe caught Lew's eye and pointed up at the tinted control-room window. "Ian Peters is on," he said. "You know him?"

"The new radiologist? No." Watkins shook his head. "I hear he's good."

"He's all right technically," Gabe said. "But he can be a real jerk sometimes."

Firbank smothered a snort and turned back to the scanner.

Working together the three men moved Lindsey—ice pack and all—onto the hard white scanner table. Her breathing had become a succession of short, sudden gasps and she had again begun to jerk her head from side to side. Watkins took the blood pressure cuff from the bottom shelf of the gurney and wrapped it around her arm. Gabe pushed open the heavy lead-shielded door and went up the three steps to the control room.

The air inside was thick with tobacco smoke. Ian Peters sat in front of a monitor showing a four-color cross-section of someone's brain. He was a stocky, abrasive little man who had trained in England during the early days of CT scanner research and felt that the machines made most of the previous practice of medicine obsolete.

"Oh, hello, Austin," he said, putting down his cigarette and swiveling his chair around. "Come in. I want to show you something *most* interesting."

"No time, Ian. We've got a very sick young lady out there. Alex Troutman's daughter. She's in hypertensive crisis. We need to find out why—and fast."

Peters tapped the tips of his short, thick fingers together, obviously displeased. "I suppose you want what you insist on calling a 'fast squash shot' for clot or bleed?"

"You got it. She's touch and go. I'm going to put on an apron and help keep her quiet for the scan. She's been thrashing around some."

Peters looked as if he'd smelled something objectionable. He raised his eyebrows like a schoolmaster about to reprimand a doltish student. "Then we'd best sedate her. It's just about impossible to get a high-quality picture—"

"Ian, we don't *need* a high-quality picture. All we need is clot or bleed. She's too sick to sedate."

"I beg your pardon, Doctor, but we do have our protocols. I'd very much—"

"Listen, Ian. This is a dear friend of mine. She's right on the edge of blowing a cerebral blood vessel. We don't have time for academic games. She's about to go out on us."

"I'd hardly call our standards of practice academic games." Peters picked up his cigarette like a piece of chalk, pointing it at Gabe's chest. "And I don't know about you being in there holding her hand during the procedure either."

"Look, Ian. Please." Gabe took a step toward him. "I don't want an argument. We just need a fast scan of this girl's brain. *Now*. Okay?"

Peters shook his head and folded his arms across his chest. He appeared to be enjoying himself. "I'm sorry," he said. "I am *not* about to violate my protocols because some part-time hot-shit media doc gets too emotionally involved."

Gabe took another step forward and stood leaning over the smaller man. He could feel himself shaking. "You want to see me get emotionally involved? You get that scan going or I'll put your head through that fucking monitor of yours."

As Gabe returned to the scanner room, Firbank was saying, "How come you got her wrapped up in all this ice, anyway? Damned if I ever seen anything like this before."

"It's an old-fashioned way to bring her blood pressure down," Watkins said, struggling to get Lindsey's head into the rubber cap built into the machine. "How the hell do you get this thing on?"

"Here. Let me do it." Firbank came around the table and with a surprising gentleness slipped Lindsey's head into the cap. "Makes me cold just to look at her. She's a real ice princess, isn't she?"

Watkins gave Gabe a worried look. "We all set?"

"All set."

Gabe put on a lead apron. Watkins and Firbank went out of the room, appearing a moment later behind the darkened observation window. Lindsey lay very still.

"It's okay, kiddo," Gabe said softly. "Hang in there just a few more minutes. Then we'll be able to give you something that will make you feel a lot better."

There was a brief silence, then the machine began to click and whir. Behind the white porcelain finish an X-ray emitter and detector moved slowly around Lindsey's head. As each slice was completed, the high white table moved a centimeter farther in, like a huge tongue being drawn slowly into the machine's round, white mouth.

It seemed to take forever. The scanner room was illuminated by banks of fluorescent lights. It seemed to Gabe as if their hypnotic blue-white vibrations were cutting away at his last remnants of energy and control. He could hear the dim, sweet voices again in the buzzing of the lights, in the whirring of the machine. They were louder now. It was all Gabe could do to keep his attention on Lindsey and on the great white machine that was sending its beam of X rays through her brain.

At last the table returned to its original position and he heard Peters's voice on the overhead speaker: *"All right, that's it."*

Gabe had the blood pressure cuff halfway around Lindsey's arm before he realized that something was wrong. It was as if he were looking down into the room from some great distance. He took her wrist and searched for the pulse but couldn't find it. *Too tired*, he thought. *Just too goddamn tired*.

He watched as a nurse came in to tell the orderly that the next patient was ready. Firbank nodded and rolled the empty stretcher back toward the table. Gabe could feel tears of frustration welling up in his eyes.

Watkins came in saying, "We'll have the scan in just a few . . ." He glanced at Gabe's face, crossed quickly to the table, and put two fingers under the angle of Lindsey's jaw. He frowned, took his stethoscope from his jacket pocket, pulled back the wet gown, and placed the diaphragm at the base of the girl's exposed left breast.

"Code Blue!" he shouted suddenly, throwing the stethoscope on the floor behind him. "She's in cardiac arrest. Come on, we've got to pump her." He leaped onto the table, dislodging a cascade of wet ice cubes. He tore the gown away, laced his fingers together on Lindsey's bare chest, and began applying external cardiac massage.

"Breathe her!" he shouted. He turned to Firbank. "Get me some oxygen and a mask and a crash cart. Call the hospital operator. Get an anesthesiologist in here."

Gabe slipped Lindsey's head out of the rubber cap, hooked his thumb over her lower teeth, and pulled her jaw all the way open. He put his mouth over hers, blowing air deep into her lungs. Her skin was cold and she offered no resistance. He took his mouth away and let Watkins's thrusting push the air out of her.

More ice spilled onto the floor. Lindsey's wide blue eyes stared up at the ceiling. She was as limp as a giant doll, her tangled hair wet and dark. Watkins dropped his weight again and again onto her chest as Gabe continued to blow air between her icy lips.

It seemed to him as if everything were moving in slow motion. Again and again he blew his breath into her, holding on to the table to keep from slipping. Gabe thought he heard a rib snap, and knew from Lew's soft curse he was right.

"Where the hell is the crash cart?" Watkins bellowed. "For Christ's sake will somebody get me those goddamn paddles?"

Then the door was thrown open, the crash cart was

pushed in, and the room was full of people, all talking at once, rushing back and forth, slipping on the ice. Someone turned on the emergency lights. An anesthesiology resident pushed Gabe away, guided an endotrachial tube down Lindsey's throat, and began breathing her with an ambu bag. It was like some old silent comedy, doctors and nurses slipping on the ice, falling, getting up, falling again.

Gabe let himself be pushed to the outside of the crowd, fell to one knee, and felt an arm around his shoulders. It was Kate. She helped him up. Her eyes glistened in the harsh light.

"Is she . . . Did she . . . ?" she asked.

"I don't know," Gabe said. He leaned against the wall. His body was shaking. His breath rattled in his throat. The voices were loud in his ears. They called on him to leave this cruel world of pain and frustration and come to them. Kate stood behind him, rubbing his shoulders, looking back at the crowd of doctors swarming over the white table.

"Poor little thing," she said.

Gabe stood with his cheek against the cool white plaster. The full weight of the past forty-eight hours came back to him: the rushed meals, the handful of serious cases, the dozens of trivial medical complaints. He hardly knew what was happening, who all these people were. He did not understand Peters's excited voice over the ceiling speakers:

"Hey, you guys. We've got a classic scan in here! Will you look at this baby, for Christ's sake? A massive intracranial bleed right in the middle of the goddamn procedure! This is a publishable case. Do you hear me? We've got ourselves a goddamn publishable case!"

5

The Bach fugue, barely audible at first, grew louder, lifting Gabe up from the depths of sleep. A soft, computerized woman's voice seemed to be speaking directly into his ear: "Dr. Gabriel Austin, this is your wake-up call. It is now six A.M. Your coffee will be ready in four minutes. Here are your top priority tasks for the day." Then, in his own voice:

My next Chronicle *column is due at two P.M.— routine Q and A's. The lead question: Drugs That Can Crash Your Sex Life. . . .*

"Gabe?" Kate's voice, full of alarm, broke through his consciousness. "What the hell is that?"

. . . Tim Jenkins at Consumer's Publishing to discuss the contract for the revised edition of Drugs and Their Side Effects.

"Gabe? Wake up. Something weird is happening."

. . . lunch meeting, medical staff of the AIDS Free Clinic . . .

He pushed himself up from beneath the pillows. "Hold on," he said. "It'll be over in a minute."

. . . meet Carlos at Stowe Lake at four P.M. for a twenty-mile training ride.

Then in the computer's voice: "This message will repeat in five minutes." The music began again.

"What the hell was that?" Kate was sitting up in the bed, her hair disheveled, her face raw with interrupted sleep. She was wearing one of his oversized gray gym shirts. She had brought him from the hospital to his apartment after Lindsey's death and had ended up staying over. They had slept together chastely.

"Just a computer program I'm testing out for Lu Jean. Sorry. I forgot it was on." He reached out for her. But she pulled away.

"You ought to warn a person for Christ's sake." She wrapped the covers tightly around her. Gabe remembered that she was not at her best in the morning.

He closed his eyes and tried to return to his dream. He had been sitting in the third row of the Lincoln High auditorium, dressed as Prince Hamlet. Lindsey was up on the stage in her Lady Macbeth costume. They had both been speaking in perfect iambic pentameter.

When she saw that he did not intend to pursue it, she sat up and turned to face him. "Really. Waking up in a strange place with that crazy thing. I almost had a heart attack."

"Sorry. Come here."

Kate sulked a moment, then moved across the bed and cuddled against him. He kissed her on the nape of her neck.

"Are you really getting up?"

The computer came to life again: "Dr. Gabriel Austin, this is your wake-up call. It is 6:05 A.M. Your coffee is ready. Here are your top-priority tasks for the day. . . ."

Kate raised her upper lip, emitting a frustrated,

half-comic growl. Gabe was already out of bed, bending over the glowing screen. The automatic coffee maker beside it had just completed its cycle.

She glared at him from the bed. "I'd forgotten about you and your early mornings. Separate bedrooms. That's an absolute requirement."

"You haven't seen the best part." He put the fresh pot of coffee on an oak tray, got a small carton of milk from the tiny refrigerator, and brought it to the bed. Kate looked down at the white china cup as if he had presented her with a wriggling insect.

"So who's this Lu Jean?" she asked.

"My office assistant. She researches my columns, handles my mail, answers my phone."

"You're sure that's all she does?"

"Relax. She's just a kid. She's going off to Swarthmore in the fall. You're sure you don't want some of this?"

"No, I'm going back to bed." She smiled, repositioned a pillow, and leaned over to kiss him lightly on the cheek. "So here we are, playing house just like an old married couple."

"Not quite."

"No, I suppose not. We'll have the unveiling later. I'm going to a medical meeting in Reno on Thursday. Maybe you could come along. Once I get done with my talk we could have a nice relaxing time."

She wrapped herself in the quilt and buried her head under the pillows. He blew her a kiss, which she never saw, then he turned out the light and carried his coffee down the hall to his office.

Lu Jean had left him an outline of proposed column ideas. A dozen letters from readers were stacked neatly on his desk, the best questions marked with yellow highlighter. Paperclipped to each letter was a copy of the journal article that would help him respond appropriately.

He opened his daily calendar and found a note from Lu Jean: "I was very sorry to hear about Lindsey. She was a good friend of mine too. The hospital called. The autopsy will be Tuesday at three P.M."

Gabe leaned forward over the desk, his hands over his eyes. He pictured Lindsey's frail body bound to the stretcher. The headache. The bleeders in her retinas. The gradually increasing blood pressure. The hospital team in their futile CPR attempt.

He blew out a long breath, turned on his computer, booted up his communications program, and directed it to link up with the National Library of Medicine. He had no energy for columns now. Marty Evans, his editor at the *Chronicle,* would scream and moan, but Gabe had given him an emergency backup piece for just such a crisis. He phoned Marty's voicemail number and left a brief message. He then set his answering machine to take all calls and turned off the bell on his phone.

Thirty seconds later he had logged on to the National Library of Medicine's medical database. He typed in the keywords *hypertensive* and *crisis*. After a few seconds he received the following response:

ITEMS	DESCRIPTION
12815	HYPERTENSIVE
4297	CRISIS
205	HYPERTENSIVE AND CRISIS

He requested title-only listings on the most recent articles that had both keywords and ran it off on his printer. He scanned the list quickly, using a yellow highlighter to mark the titles of greatest interest. He then requested full abstracts of the selected articles and printed them out. He read through the printouts, yellow marker in hand.

He was disturbed to discover that while Hyperstat (diazoxide) was still considered the treatment of choice for hypertensive crisis, there were a number of alternatives he hadn't considered. Perhaps he should have tried something else when Lindsey didn't respond. Labetalol, sodium nitroprusside, hydralazine, clonidine, camsylate, Regitine, and nitroglycerin were all established second-line drugs. There were some hot new up-and-comers, too: nifedipine, enalapril, urapidil, captopril, and co-dergocrine mesylate. He'd not heard of using them in this kind of emergency.

Gabe mentally kicked himself for not keeping up. He felt a headache coming on, as if his brain were attempting to punish itself.

Kate was still asleep when Gabe changed into his bike pants, jersey, and bike shoes and lifted his favorite street bike from the hooks in the front hall. He carried the bike down the inside staircase—what had been the rear stairs of the old Victorian house. They now led to the pharmacy storeroom.

"Hey, bub? That you?"

Larry Austin pushed open the door and peered into the storeroom. He was a big stout round-faced man like a clean-shaven Santa Claus. His bald head was surrounded by a curly white fringe that matched his short pharmacist's jacket.

"Hey, Uncle Larry. How you doing?"

"Fine. Come in for a second."

Gabe propped his bike against the wall and stepped into his uncle's office. The older man stood at the high counter, working over a display case that held two dozen pinned specimens of scarab beetles. He put an affectionate arm around Gabe's shoulders.

"So what's happening, bub? You look kind of gloomy."

"Is it that obvious?"

"Sure as hell is. What's up?"

"Tough case yesterday morning. Alex Troutman's daughter, Lindsey. She died."

"No. Gosh, I'm sorry. She was in Lu Jean's class, wasn't she?"

"Yeah."

"What did she die of?"

Gabe explained the details of the case. As he described the girl's death, he shook his head bitterly. His eyes were beginning to burn. "I keep wondering if we did the right thing. I still can't figure it out."

His uncle contorted his mouth. "You thinking about your mom?"

"No. Why?" Gabe's mother had died unexpectedly after routine gallblader surgery when Gabe was seven.

His uncle shrugged and shook his head. "Look." He put his big hands on Gabe's shoulders and shook him gently. "You did the best you could. Right?"

Gabe felt tears welling up his eyes. He nodded. "I thought so," he said. "But I guess it just wasn't good enough."

"You're a good guy, Gabe," his uncle said. "You always were. I just wish you weren't so damn hard on yourself."

Gabe nodded. He found that he could no longer

hold back his tears. He allowed himself to rest, briefly, in the bulky comfort of his uncle's arms.

Twenty minutes later he was locking his bike to a parking meter in front of the University of California School of Pharmacy. He found Gertrude Potter down in the animal room. She was sitting on a high metal stool between two rows of stainless steel cages, speaking to the large white rat she held in her lap. The air was thick with the smell of many closely bordered lives.

Gertrude wore her white hair up in a bun and looked every day of her seventy-nine years. After she had finally retired from Yale, she had been offered her own laboratory at UCSF. Gabe had followed her to San Francisco, earning his Ph.D. in pharmacology in her lab. Despite her age, and several fairly serious medical conditions, she was repeatedly voted the pharmacology students' favorite teacher. And she was still one of the most productive researchers at the medical center.

"Yes, little mousie," she was saying. "I know, I know. This cage is no fun. And this awful stuff gives you too much poops. I'm sorry, little mousie. Yes. I am sorry."

It seemed to Gabe that the rat was calmed by her touch. It looked up at her hopefully, its pink nose twitching. It hardly seemed to mind when she slipped a blunt syringe into its mouth and dribbled a measured sample of clear fluid down its throat. She leaned forward, returned the rat to its cage, and, with trembling hands, recorded the dose data in a black lab notebook.

"Hello, Gertrude. How are you?" Gabe came up beside her, crouching down so that she could see him clearly.

"Well. Gabe. How nice of you to come visit an old lady." She reached up and squeezed his hand.

"You know you should let somebody else do this," he said.

"Yes, yes. I know. This is what everybody tells me. But I like to escape down here sometimes. It is so peaceful, and I miss my mousies. Here, help me up. I'll make you a cup of tea." Gabe smiled. She had been inflicting tea on her coffee-drinking pharmacology students for nearly fifty years.

She clutched his arm on the way to the elevator, noticeably less steady than she'd been on his last visit.

"How've you been feeling?" he asked, as the elevator started up.

"Good, good, except that I get tired now and have to go home after lunch. This old age is such a strange thing. But I fool it—I get up early!"

"Your ankles look a little worse today."

"Oh, yes," she said cheerfully. "They are always worse."

"Maybe a little more diuretic?" It felt odd suggesting this to the woman who had taught him about diuretics in the first place.

She gave him an impish grin. "Well, you know, I hate to be taking these drugs."

They got off on the top floor and passed through two large laboratories where a dozen graduate students and post-docs ran centrifuges, measured radioactive isotopes, and entered data into computers. An earnest, rabbinical youth stopped to ask Gertrude a question. A shy African-American girl waited her turn.

Gabe walked down along one of the benches and

watched a tall Asian woman who was setting up an ion-exchange column. The sights and smells of glassware and reagents always brought up a powerful urge to return to this safe, insulated world of test tubes and Erlenmeyer flasks, where everything was so straightforward and you always knew exactly what you needed to do next.

Gertrude had been half-mother, half-mentor to him since his early days of medical school. It was she who had gotten him started writing his first consumer column on commonly misused drugs—for a New York women's magazine. She had made it possible for him to write a popular book on drug side effects for his doctoral thesis—a highly unusual subject for a Ph.D. dissertation. That book, *Drugs and Their Side Effects,* had launched Gabe on his present media career.

"Gabe?" It was Gertrude, calling him. He retraced his steps.

Gertrude was holding the rabbinical youth by the arm. "This is Mark Brodsky," she said. "He's a first-year pharmacy student. He has to present a brief talk on the side effects of the MAO inhibitors to his class. I thought you might help him."

Gabe smiled. "That's funny. That's one of the things I wanted to ask you about."

"Well then," she said. "We'll invite Mr. Brodsky to sit in."

Gertrude's big corner office was almost completely filled with bookshelves. Beneath a wall of bound journals and a well-thumbed reference section were two dozen copies of the current edition of her textbook, *Potter's Elements of Pharmacology.* She was notorious for giving free copies to students and friends.

Gertrude moved a pile of unopened mail from a hard leather couch and invited them both to sit down. The boy looked intensely uncomfortable.

"I hope you don't mind if I ask a lot of dumb questions," he said.

"There are no dumb questions," Gertrude said. "It is we so-called teachers who are sometimes guilty of dumb answers."

"It's really not all that complicated," Gabe said. "MAO inhibitors block the breakdown of epinephrine and norepinephrine and other similar substances which stimulate the nervous system. When their breakdown is blocked, the substances build up in the body, producing more stimulation."

The boy nodded. A hopeful look appeared in his eyes. "That makes sense," he said.

"So, let's say you took a huge overdose of an MAO inhibitor drug. You would build up more and more of these stimulating substances in your blood. Right?"

Brodsky nodded.

"So what do you think might happen?"

"Well, I guess your body would get overstimulated."

"Exactly," Gabe said. "And you'd start experiencing the symptoms of too much stimulation: restlessness, anxiety, muscle twitching, racing heartbeat, high blood pressure."

"That makes sense."

"These drugs can also interact with a wide range of foods and other drugs. When this interaction occurs, it can multiply the effects of the drug a hundred times."

The boy nodded. "Yeah, I read about that. Certain drugs and certain foods. So why would you want to use these drugs at all, if they're so dangerous?''

Gabe smiled. "There's some risk in taking *any* drug. But sometimes the potential benefits of a drug are so great and the condition is so serious that it's worth the risk.''

Gertrude gave the boy a copy of her textbook. After he left, she poured two cups of tea at her small lab bench. "Look,'' she said. "Tea bags. I have become an American at last. My hands shake too much. I broke three teapots. *Three.*'' She laughed at her own foolishness. "So. What can I help you with?'' she said. "Something for that wonderful column of yours?''

"No. It's about a patient.'' He gave her a quick summary of what had happened to Lindsey.

"So you think she died of a stroke?'' she said.

"Yes. But we don't know what caused it.''

Gertrude settled herself in her leather desk chair, the steaming mug in her hands. "Well, could it perhaps have been a congenital defect or a ruptured cerebral aneurysm?''

Gabe shook his head. "They'll be looking for that at the autopsy, but that wouldn't explain the increase in blood pressure.''

"Well, there is always our old friend the pheochromocytoma, of which the internists are so fond.'' A pheochromocytoma is an extremely rare tumor of the kidney that can produce high blood pressure.

"Possible, but unlikely. They'll look for that too.''

"Or perhaps you are thinking of an MAO inhibitor reaction? Was she taking any MAO inhibitor drugs?''

"Apparently not. But she was taking birth control pills. And she was a smoker.''

Gertrude nodded. "You are thinking perhaps of the Jennifer Cross case?"

"Maybe." Gabe nodded.

"Any other drugs involved?"

"Not according to her mother."

"Mothers do not always know. The MAO drugs are used for a wide variety of psychiatric problems these days. A seventeen-year-old girl might go to a doctor on her own. Or get some pills from a friend. You did a blood test for MAO inhibitor activity?"

Gabe shook his head. "We don't have that at our hospital. Could you do it here if I brought in a sample?"

"Yes, of course. We do it for our mousies all the time," she said. "We cannot give you a precise level, or the specific drugs involved, but sure, we could tell you yes or no." Her brown eyes twinkled. "Now we will have one more cup of tea and you will tell me all about our old friend Kate Reiley, who is all over the sports pages these last few months."

6

The emergency room at St. Catherine's was almost deserted. The day secretary was helping a tall woman in a leg cast walk back to X ray. The duty doc, Chris Stevens, was in cubicle 6, talking to a woman with a crying baby. Elsa and Lucille were in the staff room, drinking coffee. Gabe used the secretary's phone to call Charlie Cusick, downstairs, then walked back to cubicle 3.

There were clean green sheets on the examining table. The stainless steel counters and white cabinets glistened. He pulled the supply cabinet away from the wall and found a dozen blood tubes taped to the back, all bearing the names of his former patients. He located the tube with Lindsey's name on it, wrapped it in a paper towel, and put it in a cardboard specimen container. He dropped the others into the shiny white trash receptacle.

He found Charlie Cusick at the dissecting table at the back of the pathology laboratory, talking into a microphone that hung from the ceiling. He was using a large butcher knife to cut a kidney into half-inch slices. Melissa Lyons, a fourth-year medical student at UC, stood a few feet away, her arms folded, looking down at the floor. She had done an ER rotation with Gabe the previous year.

". . . no infarcts, tumors, or congenital abnormalities were seen, stop." Cusick took his foot off the pedal, glaring across at Gabe. "About time you showed up," he said. "I thought you wanted to see this for Christ's sake."

"Hey, Charlie. Sorry I'm late." Gabe had timed his arrival to miss the first part of the procedure: the gross examination of the body, the long, Y-shaped incision running from shoulders to pubis, and the removal of the organs. He had, on several previous occasions, attempted to explain to Cusick that there were matters of personal sensibility involved.

"Hey, Melissa," he said. "How you making out with this guy?" He saw at once that it was the wrong thing to say.

"Hi, Dr. Austin." She did not meet his eyes. "Fine, just fine." Her words were unconvincing. She glanced across at Cusick, made sure he wasn't looking, and rolled her eyes up at the ceiling.

Cusick nodded down at the cutting board. "This is your patient here." He stepped on the pedal again. "The renal arteries showed minimal signs of atherosclerotic plaques, stop. There were multitudinous superficial pinpoint hemorrhages throughout the parenchymal tissue. There were no signs of calcifications, stones, or other abnormalities in the collecting system, stop." He put down the knife, picked up the cutting board, and slid the slices of kidney tissue into a shallow glass specimen dish.

"You busted one of her ribs."

"Yeah, we figured," Gabe said. Even the most conscientious doctors will occasionally fracture a patient's rib during a resuscitation attempt. "You didn't see any sign of a pheochromocytoma?"

Cusick snorted and shook his head. "I've seen maybe two of those in my whole career. I think that's something they made up over at the medical school. Come on, what are you waiting for?" He jabbed his thumb toward a peg that held a black rubber apron. Gabe put on the apron and pulled on a pair of rubber gloves. When he returned, Cusick was using the knee control to turn on the water in the sink. He washed off the cutting board and rinsed his rubber-gloved hands. "Miss Lyons, tell Dr. Austin about the case we just did."

Melissa cleared her throat and began presenting the findings in a low voice: "The patient was a well-developed, well-nourished seventeen-year-old white female with superficial contusions of the chest. Findings on gross exam were unremarkable except for the fractured rib and multiple hemorrhages in various organs. There was some mild damage to the muscle of the heart. The stomach contents were sent to the lab for analysis. Gross exam of the brain revealed a number of pinpoint hemorrhages on the superficial aspect of the cerebral cortex. Further examination was postponed pending proper tissue preparation."

"Got it right here," Cusick said. He took the lid off a white metal bucket, reached in with his gloved hands, lifted out a quivering whitish mass the size of a small melon, and set it on the wet cutting board. The cloudy fixative fluid ran down the drainage grooves into the sink.

"Like Miss Lyons says, this thing had superficial bleeders up the wazoo. There was a clot as big as an egg on the brain stem. We'll see what's inside." He picked up a long, clean knife and began to slice through the soft tissue.

There was a heavy thump behind them. Gabe

turned and saw that Melissa had gone down on one knee. She was leaning against a glass case that held a display of fetal abnormalities.

Cusick muttered a curse. "Is she going out on me again?" He growled. "Gabe, get her out of here, will you? I'm two cases behind as it is." Gabe stripped off his gloves, went around the table, and put a hand on the girl's shoulder.

"It's okay," he said. "Come on, let's go outside for a minute." He got an arm around her waist and helped her up. Her lower lip was trembling. They made their way out of the room a step at a time.

"Dammit anyway," she said, as he lowered her onto one of the straight chairs in the hall. "I was fine for the autopsy itself. I thought . . ."

"It's okay," Gabe said, patting her shoulder. "I did the same thing when I was a med student. A lot of us did. You get used to it eventually."

She shook her head. "It's not the procedure," she said. "It's *him*. He is *such* a pig. Why does he get away with it? Why?"

"Because he's a good pathologist," Gabe said. "He could walk out of here tomorrow and get a job at any hospital in town. There are a lot of others who are just as bad. At least he doesn't see patients. You okay now?"

"I . . . I think so."

"Good. You just wait out here for a little bit. You'll be fine. I need to go back."

She grasped his hand and held it with a desperate strength. He watched the shudder go through her body. It started in her jaw and passed down through her shoulders.

"Sometimes I'm afraid that's what's going to happen to me," she said. "What do you have to do to keep yourself from turning into an asshole like Charlie Cusick?''

By the time Gabe got back inside, Cusick had sliced the brain into uniform slices and was examining them with a hand lens. Without looking up from the table he said, "I hope you had better luck with her than I did."

"What are you talking about?" Gabe pulled on his gloves and stepped up to the counter.

"Don't play cute with me," Cusick said. "I saw her following you around when she was on your rotation. I know you were banging her."

Gabe laughed. "You've got to be kidding, Charlie. I don't get involved with my medical students."

Cusick appeared not to hear. "You goddamn ER guys have all the luck. Glamor. Excitement. What do we have down here? Goddamn dead bodies and formaldehyde. So tell me: was she any good?"

"You're way off base, Doctor."

"You should hear how she talks about you for Christ's sake."

"I was nice to her, Charlie. You really ought to try it sometime."

"I'll be as nice as she likes, if she'd give me half a chance."

Gabe had to close his eyes and look away for a minute, reminding himself why he had come. He drew a deep breath and looked down at the specimen. "So what have we got?" he asked. "Clot or bleed?"

Cusick poked at a bit of tissue with a probe. "The cerebral vessels are distended as hell. There's been massive bleeding into the brain at several locations. The clots we found are all postmortem stuff."

"So it wasn't the Pill."

"Not likely."

"There was no head injury?"

"No."

"No brain tumor? No hormone-secreting tumors? No aneurysms or congenital defects?"

"What's the matter, you been reading a pathology book or something?" Cusick scratched his temple with the inside of his gloved wrist. "There's none of that shit. So listen. Put in a good word for me, will you? She likes you." He slid the specimens into a basin of fixative to prepare them for microscopic analysis.

"So what do you think?" Gabe asked.

"The primary lesion, you mean? Well, I'll go ahead and do the microscopics, but it's not going to tell us anything. I'd say you've got yourself a world-class case of malignant hypertension of nonanatomic origin."

"So you're telling me it was some kind of a toxic reaction."

Cusick shrugged. "That's about what's left. We'll have the lab report on the stomach contents on Wednesday. So do me a favor. Go see if that hostile little twit is ready to come back in here and help me clean up."

7

Gabe left the hospital a little after five o'clock. He headed west on Stanyan Street, catching the evening rush hour. He inched his old Volvo station wagon through the fog drifting in from the ocean. It took him twenty minutes to cover the twelve blocks to his apartment.

He punched in the security code deactivating the building's alarm, let himself in at the pharmacy's back door, and went up the stairs. His housekeeper had been in during the day. He could smell a faint lemon scent from the cleaning supplies she used.

Lu Jean had left a list of his calls. There was one from Kate. He reached her answering machine and left what he hoped was a subtly romantic message. He decided that the others could wait until later.

He stood on tiptoe to reach the cabinet over the sink, and got down the big bottle of Southern Comfort that had been left after a party months ago. Gabe rarely drank hard liquor. He reminded himself that there was a time for everything.

He filled his glass, carried it into the living room, and opened the high Victorian bay window that looked over Clayton Street. He knelt on the couch, sipping his drink and looking out at the darkening sky.

Rain was coming down in earnest now. He looked at the neon sign in the dry cleaner's window across the street, that old, soft neon they never used anymore. He remembered looking out this window at the old pharmacy sign, years ago, when he lived here with his mother and father. It had those same, soft colors. His mother had loved that old sign as much as he did. But his uncle's business partner had pressured him to replace it with a big, blaring Vegas–style plastic sign with standard fluorescent tubes that could be easily replaced.

He closed the window and carried his drink into the big front bedroom that served as his office. Lu Jean had sorted his mail into a row of labeled baskets—Urgent, Good Stuff, Reader Mail, Financial, Medical Journals, and Throwaways. There was nothing in the Urgent box and he did not feel up to looking at the other piles. He picked up the red rubber mousepad from his desk and sailed it harmlessly across the room.

As if that was her cue, the cat door clattered and Princess came trotting in. She stopped in the doorway, peering up at him curiously. He bent down, balancing his drink on his knee, and scratched under her chin. She closed her eyes, arched her back, and emitted a soft sound that had elements of a growl, a purr, and a questioning meow. He picked her up, carried her to the couch, and held her in his lap, scratching the top of her head and watching the golden strands of fur adhere to his dark gray slacks.

He fed the cat, poured himself another drink, and carried it back to the office. The digital readout on his phone machine told him that he had received one call between the time Lu Jean had left and he had arrived.

"Hi, Gabe. This is Margaret Troutman. . . . I just got a call from one of Lindsey's friends. . . . Oh, Jesus, Gabe. Those sweet kids are going to have a memorial service over at the school tonight. Seven o'clock in the Lincoln High auditorium. Sally Powers called and asked me specially if I'd invite you. She feels it's very important for you to be there. There was a suicide at the school last week and some of the kids are worried that Lindsey might have killed herself. We'd love it if you could come and set them straight. I know this is pretty short notice. Hope you can make it. Bye-bye."

Gabe left his car in the teachers' parking lot and climbed the familiar stairs to the Lincoln High auditorium. The smell of the place brought back a flood of old memories—the long, dull high school assemblies, the theater productions of his own thespian days, and, most recently, the productions in which Lindsey had the starring role.

Twenty-five or thirty people, most of them students, had gathered on the stage. They were standing in a big circle, holding hands. He spotted Margaret and her husband Alex, Sally Powers, Lu Jean, and Lindsey's boyfriend Bobby. He recognized a few of the others from the plays.

Lu Jean spotted him and waved. He hurried down the aisle and up the echoing flight of steps to the stage. Sally and Margaret dropped hands and welcomed him into the circle.

"Glad you could make it," Sally said. She was a funny, upbeat little dynamo of a woman who was a second mother to the kids in her drama class. Margaret nodded and squeezed Gabe's hand. She was crying, looking down at the pieces of tape on the floor that had marked the stage movements for Lindsey and the others. Gabe nodded across at Alex, Lindsey's father, tall and blond, who stood glum and silent in his grief. He nodded a greeting across the circle at Lu Jean, a gangly young woman in an olive drab T-shirt with long, floppy sleeves, and to Bobby, the blond boy on Sally's left. The other students inspected Gabe politely. A face here and there was glistening with tears.

Sally began again. "Lindsey was one of the most alive, vital people I've ever known," she said. "And she was such a wonderful young actress. She and Bobby had been accepted to the theater program at NYU for next year." Bobby was looking down at his black-and-white running shoes.

"She once told me she never felt as alive as when she was onstage," Sally said. "It was a real gift to have her here with us. I don't think anyone who ever saw her work will ever forget her. And I know that the time she spent with us meant a lot to her."

There was a ripple of agreement. A tall, red-haired girl with tears running down her cheeks raised her hand.

"Yes, Hillary?"

"What I remember most was the way she helped me with that little nothing part I had in our first play last year. I'd never been onstage before and I was afraid I'd start shaking or something. Lindsey stayed late with me every night for the last two weeks, helping me through my part. God, I'm really going to miss her."

Several other members of the class shared their memories of Lindsey. When they were finished, Sally brought the focus around to Gabe.

"Most of you know Dr. Gabe Austin. Gabe was

the doctor who took care of Lindsey at the hospital. Several of you have expressed concern about the way Lindsey died. Alex and Margaret and I have asked Gabe to explain exactly what caused Lindsey's death so you'll all understand.''

Gabe felt a tingling in his arms and shoulders. They were waiting. He felt hopelessly inadequate to the task. He hadn't been able to save Lindsey. He didn't even really know how she had died. He cleared his throat.

"First of all," he said, "I want to assure you all that there is nothing whatsoever to suggest that Lindsey took her own life." Heads nodded. Whispers broke out on all sides.

"She died as the result of a massive increase in her blood pressure. Doctors call this hypertensive crisis. It's a condition in which the blood pressure keeps going up and up. We did everything we could to bring her pressure down." He paused to shake his head, remembering the feel of Lindsey's frail, trembling body under his hands.

"The actual cause of death was apparently a stroke—a burst blood vessel in the brain. It's a very unusual case. We still don't really understand what caused it. We may never know. But I can assure you that Lindsey did *not* do anything to harm herself."

There was a murmur of relief all around. Sally nodded and squeezed his hand.

"Thank you, Gabe," she said. "We all appreciate your coming here to share that with us. And now, if no one has anything more to say, I thought it would be a fitting memorial if we watched the video of the final scene from *Our Town*. This sequence seems all too appropriate, given the events of the last few days.

"As you'll remember, Emily has just died in childbirth and is taking her place among the other deceased residents of Grover's Corners in the big cemetery on the hill. I think the scene pretty much speaks for itself.'' She waved up at the projection booth. The stage lights dimmed. The video filled the screen above them.

Lindsey was dressed in a delicate white lace frock. Her shoulders were bare. She was lit by a single, pinpoint spotlight. The stage manager, played by Bobby in a battered top hat, was escorting her away from the black umbrellas of her funeral and toward the three nervous rows of teenagers in gray hair and beards sitting stiffly in their folding chairs, representing the deceased former citizens of the town.

Gabe felt a lump rising in his throat as Lindsey offered her last goodbyes to Grover's Corners. To clocks ticking. To food and coffee and Mama's sunflowers. She asked Bobby if anyone was really aware of this incredible life we live, if they were able to stay conscious every minute.

"No," he replied. "The saints and poets, maybe."

Lindsey shook her head and made her way back up the plywood hill to her folding-chair grave. A tall, frail youth with wispy chinwhiskers pushed himself up, leaned on his cane, and looked over at her accusingly.

He delivered an angry diatribe against the living, explaining how they moved about in a cloud of ignorance, trampling on the feelings of those around them. How they wasted their time as if they expected to live forever. How they dozed through their lives, driven by one self-centered passion after another. "Now you know," he concluded. "Now you know."

As he was speaking, a handsome youth playing Emily's husband came slowly up the hill. As he reached Emily's grave he threw himself at her feet. Lindsey looked down at him as if from a great distance. She turned to the stout, nervous, gray-wigged girl on the chair beside her.

"Mrs. Gibbs?" she said. "They don't understand. Do they?"

The heavy girl shook her head sadly and took Lindsey's hand. "No, dear," she said. "They just don't understand."

8

At one o'clock that Thursday afternoon, Gabe and Kate were standing in a long line at gate 26 at San Francisco Airport, waiting to get boarding passes for the Reno shuttle. Kate was giving a paper at the Western Medical Association's annual meeting and had invited him to come along.

Gabe's scruffy suit bag stood out in marked contrast to Kate's matching black leather carry-on and briefcase. He admired her smart jacket and skirt, her soft leather boots. He wondered how her upper body looked under her clothes. She had—understandably enough—become extremely shy since her mastectomy. He would have to be very patient. And very gentle.

Kate was reading over the notes for her talk. Some of the other Reno passengers had already started celebrating. The couple behind them was toasting their upcoming vacation with a bottle in a brown paper bag. Their three young boys, all wearing Mickey Mouse hats, bumped into people as they chased one another in a game of You're It.

Gabe wondered at how much Kate had changed since that first August day in 1976. He'd been crossing the lobby of the Harkness Medical Student Dormitory when he heard the notes of Bach's *Chromatic Fantasy and Fugue*, played on a steel-stringed guitar.

He'd found her in the next room, a pretty, long-haired girl with a round, Irish face. She was curled up on the sofa, finger-picking the melody on a battered old Martin, wearing running shoes, a faded pair of jeans, and a University of Michigan track T-shirt. It was a wild, exalted piece, full of exuberant feeling. But she kept it under perfect control.

She was married to Andy, a bearded neurology resident. They had come out from Ann Arbor the month before and were living in a cramped double in the married students' quarters. Gabe had a friend at the law school who had rented a big rambling place out near the Yale Bowl and was looking for roommates. Three days later, they all moved into the Edgewood Avenue house.

Kate became very involved in the New Haven women's movement and had become a key member of YCWM, the Yale Committee for Women in Medicine. Gabe and Kate frequently sat together in the med school lecture halls. She had felt very insecure at first, but as the months passed, Gabe watched her confidence increase. Neither of them could believe that most of their classmates wore coats and ties and dresses to class, as if adopting a certain dress code were just as important a part of their medical training as learning about the bones of the hand or the names and functions of the twelve cranial nerves. Andy wore an endless succession of rumpled green scrubs and looked exactly the same at home as he did at the hospital.

Halfway through their sophomore year, Andy came home to announce that he was getting a divorce. He moved out that evening, giving no satisfactory explanation. He was reasonable, kind, and un-approachable.

Three months after Andy had left, Gabe and Kate became lovers. They kept their separate rooms, but had considered themselves a committed couple from then on.

Gabe took to the monkish routine of lectures, labs, and study like a man born to the task. But this dry academic approach to medicine was difficult for Kate. She became very involved in an effort to put women's athletics on an even footing with the men's program. She had been a middle-distance runner at the University of Michigan and was invited to work out with the Yale women's track team. Even then, out of shape and carrying twenty extra pounds, she could run like the wind. She began serious training, shed most of her excess weight, and began to compete in local AAU track meets. The demands of her training and her political work left her little time for her studies. At the end of her sophomore year, she failed Part 1 of the National Medical Board examinations.

An unusually high number of women had failed the exam and several conservative members of the Yale faculty were calling for a cutback in female admissions. Then, just as Kate was repeating several courses and studying to take the exam again, Gabe was assigned to a prestigious subinternship at a hospital in Hartford. It was a huge honor, but it required him to be away for days at a time. It was a difficult period for Kate. He should have turned down the subinternship and helped Kate through her time of need. Gabe was convinced that it was his failure to do so that had led to their split. He saw now, in retrospect, how self-centered he had been.

He had never since been able to find a relationship that felt so natural, so right. During his time with Kate he was as happy as he had ever been.

Gabe was surprised to find that they had seats in the first-class section. The flight steward took their coats and their order for drinks. Gabe's Heineken and Kate's white wine were on their tray tables within minutes.

"So this is how the executive class flies," he said.

"This is it," she said. She set her glass down and stretched her arms high above her head.

"So who is it you're working for now?" he said. "You never did say. Is it some big secret or what?"

"I really don't want to talk about work right now," Kate said, shaking her head. She reached across the armrest to take his hand. "Indulge me. Okay?"

"Hey." He shrugged. "I'm easy. But curious." The steward pulled the big door closed and the plane began to move away from the gate.

"I'll tell you soon. I promise." She squeezed his hand. "So how was the autopsy?"

He shook his head, sipping at his beer. "A hard one," he said. He told her about it and the memorial service. "I talked to one of her girlfriends afterward," he said. "She told me Lindsey would sometimes make herself vomit after a big meal."

"You'd be surprised how many girls her age are bulimic," Kate said. "But that wouldn't cause high blood pressure, would it?"

"Not directly. But there's an antidepressant called phenelzine that's sometimes used to treat bulimia. It's not used much because it can produce an MAO-inhibitor reaction. I realize it's kind of grabbing at straws, but I've got to track down every possibility.''

"So it wasn't the Pill?" Kate said.

"No. It wasn't the Pill. There was no head injury. No brain tumor. No hormone-secreting tumors. No congenital abnormalities.''

"So what was it then?"

Gabe shook his head and finished his beer. "That's what we're still trying to find out.''

"Oh, babes. Why can't you just let it go? This whole business is turning into an obsession.''

"Yes. I realize that.''

"You really have a thing for this girl, don't you.''

He nodded. "I used to dream she was my daughter.''

"If it's that important, you've got to go for it Gabe. Do whatever it takes.'' She squeezed his hand again. They looked out the window as the jet turned onto the runway and the engines went to full power. The jet gathered speed, rocked slightly from side to side. Then they were pressed back into their seats as the plane lifted sharply into the air.

The Reno Hilton stands out among the gaudy jumble of hotel-casinos like a tweedy matron in a row of hookers. It's where people stay when they want to convince themselves they haven't come to town to gamble.

But the facade is only skin-deep. There are a hundred slot machines within fifty feet of the casino entrance. Kate stopped, astounded by the scene, blocking a party of chattering white-haired ladies dressed as if for church. A man in red coveralls walked by, wheeling a heavy metal cart stacked with rolls of coins. A uniformed guard moved silently beside him.

A young woman in an astonishingly skimpy outfit came up to Gabe, looked into his eyes with a guileless innocence, welcomed him to the casino, and offered him a coupon good for a complimentary cocktail. She was a fresh-faced girl of twenty with a fine, long neck and bright green eyes. Her delicately chiseled cheekbones were lightly beaded with sweat. She moved on to a party of three elderly men in cowboy boots. Gabe and Kate watched as she repeated her performance.

"I'm not sure I'm ready for this," Kate said.

"Never been to Reno before?"

"No. And I'm not sure I'm coming back real soon." She slipped her hand through his arm in a possessive gesture. "Really," she said. "Can you *believe* this place?"

"We need to go all the way across the casino and up the escalator," he said. She gripped his hand tightly and they made their way down the aisle between two curving rows of slot machines. Suddenly bells began to ring, lights began to flash, and two young women wearing the same minimal costumes came running up to present a bald man in a tan leisure suit with a big tub of quarters. He set it down on a high stool and began feeding the coins back into the machine.

It was quieter upstairs, the murmur of the casino floor softened by the thick carpet and large tapestries depicting desert and mountain scenes. The registration area was full of doctors with plastic name tags. They were clapping one another's shoulders and whispering in one another's ears, as wide-eyed as a class of Sunday-school children let out of church on a sunny morning.

The desk clerk was a gracious young blond woman

with an impressive tan. "Oh, yes. Dr. Austin," she said. "There's a message for you."

Gabe opened the envelope. His face broke into a smile. "It's from Michael Jefferson. He's got a booth in the exhibit area downstairs. He wants me to stop by."

The desk clerk checked Gabe into his modest fourth-floor single. Her eyes lit up when she found that Kate was booked into a suite on the concierge floor.

"Yes, the Sierra Suite. You'll just love it," she assured her. "It's certainly where *I'll* stay as soon as I can afford it." She seemed to have no doubts that such a time lay just around the corner. A veteran bellman with no such illusions loaded their bags on a cart and took them up in the elevator.

"The concierge floor?" Gabe asked, as they went up.

Kate was embarrassed. "My new employer," she said. "They're still giving me the red carpet treatment." The look in her eye kept Gabe from asking any further questions.

They stopped by his room to drop off his bags, then continued on to Kate's penthouse suite, a complex of large, airy rooms with oak paneling and long leather couches. There were a dozen red roses in a vase on the coffee table, a color TV in the bathroom, and a fully stocked minibar. The bellman set out Kate's bags, adjusted the air conditioner, demonstrated the remote control for the TV, and recommended several dishes from the room service menu. She gave him a ten-dollar bill.

Gabe drew back the drapes and looked out at the glowing silhouette of the Sierras in the distance. He went over to examine the mahogany rolltop desk. According to the engraved brass plate, it had belonged to a nineteenth-century Supreme Court justice.

"Nice pad," he said.

"It's a bit of a mixed blessing," Kate said, pouring herself a glassful of club soda. "The corporate world is different."

"Different good or different bad?"

"Just . . . different." She had taken off her jacket and stood at the mirror, fussing with her hair, her chest rising and falling under her silk blouse with the movement of her arms.

"Michael Jefferson," she said, smiling. "I always liked Michael. He was very nice to me."

"He liked you because you were a fighter," Gabe said.

"He was one of the few people who did. Medical school does a pretty good job of making a strong, independent woman feel like a freak."

"It was hard for all of us," he said. He put his arms around her waist and nuzzled in her hair. She continued to look at her reflection. "But you've got it together now. The running. Your wellness program. The people at your company obviously think a lot of you."

"It's nothing personal. They like the idea of having a world-class runner on staff," she said. "They don't like women much. I get the feeling I'm going to have to play the part, not make waves, and cover my ass every goddamn minute." She leaned her head back against his shoulder, rolling it back and forth.

"I'm a wreck," she said. "Can you believe I'm supposed to be running the San Francisco Women's Marathon next week."

"Sure. I read all about it in the *Chronicle*."

"There's a lot of pressure on me to win. But I'm running against Katrina Maritova. I've never beaten her. I'm not sure I can. But the company is already talking about doing this big victory tour. I'm supposed to go around to fifteen cities in three weeks as a sort of goodwill ambassador. Do you know I've actually been taking medication for anxiety this last few weeks? I've been having rapid heartbeats. I've been hyperventilating. Do you remember how we used to joke about *globus hystericus* on our psychiatry clerkship? Well it's no joke, sweetie. I've been having it on and off." *Globus hystericus* is the subjective sensation of a lump in the throat and is frequently seen in cases of intense anxiety.

He nodded. "Anything I can do to help?"

"There *is* something. You can ride along with me on your bike during the race. Toss me water bottles and such. I've got all the gear."

"I'd be honored."

"You mean it?"

"Sure."

She smiled. "That'd be nice."

"We all need support," he said. "Even a tough chick like you."

"*Especially* tough women like me. Because we've just learned to *pretend* we're tough, that's all. Men with those kinds of defenses actually believe they really *are* tough." She smiled down into her glass.

"Let me be frank, Gabe. I've got a lot of liabilities as a romantic partner. I'm a one-tit wonder. I'm not very good at compromising. I'm not always as diplomatic as I could be. I keep this ridiculous training schedule. And there aren't that many eligible men out there in the first place. Not in the Bay Area at least. Oh, Christ. I didn't want to cry."

"Hey," he said, putting his arms around her. "You're among friends."

"I *do* feel you're my friend. I always have. Even

through the worst of it. Sometimes I want to just curl up with you under the covers and have you take care of me. Like you did after Andy left."

"I could get into that." He kissed her.

She put her hands on the sides of his face and looked into his eyes for a long time.

"Christ," she said. "I've missed you."

She stood on tiptoe to kiss him, then slipped off his jacket and began to unbutton his shirt. She shook her head, laughed, and pressed her cheek against his bare chest. She locked her hands behind his waist and leaned back to look up at him.

"See? I can still get all mushy. Just like the old days."

"The old days were not so bad," he said. He reached down to touch her face. He felt her shiver as he traced the line of her neck with his fingertips. Her body was limber and fit under his hands. She was like some warm, playful jungle cat, purring against him.

She took his hand and led him through the open French doors into the bedroom. And neither of them said anything else for a long time.

9

Gabe was awakened by a soft whirring sound. He was lying in the largest king-sized bed he had ever seen. Kate was sitting on the far corner. She had pulled back the drapes, and the last tones of sunset filled the bedroom, lighting her face with a soft golden glow.

He watched her fondly across the bed. She was wearing her running outfit and drying her hair with a tiny hair drier. It seemed as if they had never been apart. He remembered the way she had always experienced a burst of manic energy after making love.

"Back to reality, sweetie." She pulled the plug on the machine, skipped across the room, and leaped back onto the bed beside him. "So. Did you notice anything?"

"Your new breast, you mean? No, not really," he said. She had pulled on an oversized T-shirt before getting into bed.

"It's pretty good in the dark," she said. "We'll have the full unveiling later when we're not so rushed. I've got to run. Literally. This close to a race, I really can't afford to miss a day." She worked at her hair with a tortoiseshell brush. "The company's hosting a dinner at Chez Nous tonight. It's a really good French restaurant. I'd love it if you'd come."

"Sure. I might find out who the hell you're working for."

"Oh, shit. Right. I guess we need to have that conversation right now." She got off the bed, poured herself another club soda, and came back to sit beside him. "The express version, right? No arguments. I tell you and I'm out of here. We can discuss it later. Agreed?"

"All right, dammit. Agreed."

She nodded. "Okay. Ta-da." She let out a deep breath. "I'm running the fitness program up at Kimberley Labs."

"Ed Elias's program?"

"That's the one."

"You're kidding." Kimberley Labs was, in Gabe's estimation, one of the most predatory drug companies in the country. He had frequently criticized the company—its CEO, its sales tactics, and its products—in his newspaper column. He squinted out at the horizon, the faint band of deep red glowing above the long strip of dark mountains. He opened his mouth to speak. Kate held up a hand.

"You're not kidding," he said.

"You promised."

"Yeah, I know, but, Kate, Kimberley Labs. Ed Elias . . ." He made a face and brought the covers up over his head.

"Have you ever met him?"

Gabe came up from beneath the blanket. "No. I've tried to get an interview with him half a dozen times. He's always turned me down flat."

"I'll see what I can do. You may be surprised to find that he's really a pretty decent guy."

"Ed Elias," Gabe said. "God help us."

"There's more. It gets worse." She rolled the glass between her palms, bending over to let the beads of condensation fall to the carpet. "I was going out with Ed for a while. I was consulting for the company for about nine months before I moved out here. Their whole program is based on the one I developed at the University of Michigan. He used to fly out to see me in Ann Arbor."

"You were sleeping with this guy? Christ, Kate, he must be in his sixties."

She shrugged. "I'm a big girl, Gabe. I'd just split up with Russell. Ed was a real gentleman. And it was never all that serious. I put an end to it the day I realized he wasn't kidding about offering me the job."

"Oh boy . . ."

"Look, I'm trying to be straight, okay? You want to give me a chance?" She closed her eyes briefly, as if collecting her thoughts.

"For some reason I don't understand, Ed is convinced I hung the moon," she said. "He not only wants me to run his new wellness program, he wants me to be the voice and face for the company."

"Sure. You're going to be the Michael Jordan of the pharmaceutical industry."

She blushed and nodded. "Something like that. He's also nominated me to be the first woman on Kimberley's board of directors."

Gabe shook his head. "He wants you for your publicity value, baby. You're hot this month. Next year it'll be somebody else."

"I know. I'm not counting on anything long-term. But this fits in perfectly with my personal agenda."

Gabe smiled. " 'Baby, I'm gonna make you a star.' "

The color rose in her face. "It's not like that at

all," she insisted. "It's a straight business deal. I'm going into it with my eyes wide open. After all, I did break off with him. And I waited for three months after I did to come see you."

"But you're still working for him," Gabe said. "And you sound like you think he's a great guy."

"I can be very critical of Ed," Kate said. "I know him pretty well by now. But I do admire the man. He has this idea he wants to talk to you about. I'm really excited about it too. For your sake as well as the company's. But all that just sort of confuses things, because I wanted to see you, too, for reasons of my own." She swallowed the rest of the club soda and ran her finger around the rim of the empty glass.

"Because in spite of the fact that you can be an insensitive, distant, macho, self-involved workaholic, I happen to like you quite a bit. And respect you. You know what a moody bitch I can be. And you don't fall apart when I get angry. In my experience, that's pretty rare in a man."

He saw the color rising in her cheeks. She looked flushed and relieved, like a woman who has completed a difficult mission. She glanced at her watch, put down her glass, and punched him lightly on the shoulder.

"Don't let it go to your head," she said, standing up. "And now I've really *got* to go run. It's suit and tie tonight. I'll meet you down at Michael's booth at seven-thirty. Okay?" She paused with one hand on the door, blowing him a kiss.

"All right," he said. "You're a crazy woman, you know."

"That's right. And don't you forget it." She fluttered her lashes, gave him an elaborate wink, and pulled the door closed behind her.

10

Gabe found himself walking through the exhibit area with a huge smile on his face. He supposed it was some combination of postcoital high and the grand commercial spectacle laid out before him: space-age splints and bandages, sparkling surgical equipment, motor-driven examination tables, X-ray machines, IV fluids in bags and bottles, and enough drugs to stock a dozen pharmacies.

Workmen on scaffolds were hanging long garlands of red and white crepe paper from the ceiling. An electric forklift with white canvas tire covers drove past carrying an automated examining table the size of a small Mercedes.

This was the kind of scene Gabe would usually criticize in his writing, yet here he was, all dressed up in his best Brooks Brothers suit, wandering through the display areas looking for drug-company freebies. The whole thing struck him as quite ridiculous.

The exhibit area occupied the entire hotel ballroom and spilled over into an adjacent reception hall. Gabe walked up and down the rows, watching the representatives of a hundred companies arranging their wares. As he was walking past a half-assembled booth, he spotted a thin, sleek man in tie and shirtsleeves lying on his back beneath a long folding table that held six laptop computers. He was connecting a heavy electrical cable to a black plastic outlet box.

"Hey there, Professor. How's it hanging?" Gabe said.

"Mmm? Say what?" Michael Jefferson peered up from under the table, a row of red and yellow wire connectors in his teeth. "Gabe Austin. Well I'll be damned." He spat the connectors into his hand, his thin, ebony face breaking into a smile. He had a flat-top Afro, white, even teeth, and a neatly trimmed beard. He stood up and pumped Gabe's hand.

"My man. How you doing?" he said. "I guess that last quake didn't get your ass after all." He rested his weight on the edge of the computer table. He was wearing a custom-tailored white shirt with a monogram on the pocket. The jacket of his sleek Italian suit hung over the back of a folding chair.

"We came through all right," Gabe said. "I got your note. How'd you know I was here?"

"Virginia Davis said she saw you and Kate Reiley at the airport." Michael raised his eyebrows, twisting his face into a mask of incredulous amazement. "So what gives? You two old flames getting back together?"

"Could be." Gabe smiled and shrugged. "So far, so good. She's just moved out to San Francisco."

"So I heard. I've been reading all about her. She had breast cancer or something, didn't she?"

"Yeah. A couple of years ago. She appears to have licked it."

"I guess. She's been really kicking ass on the women's marathon circuit. Why was she wasting herself trying to do medicine, anyway?"

"You'll have to ask her that," Gabe said. "So how

about you, Michael? You still playing the field or you got somebody serious?"

"Oh, man." Jefferson smiled and shook his head. "I may have slowed down a little, but I'm still a kid in the candy store when it comes to these California ladies. I mean to tell you, Southern California women . . . Mmmmm . . . I just have to force myself to be . . . you know, selective."

Gabe looked back toward the booth. "So what's all this?"

"My new software. Here. Check this out." He picked up his jacket, turning the lapel so that Gabe could read his name tag.

```
MICHAEL ALLEN JEFFERSON, M.D.
HIPPOCRATES MEDICAL SYSTEMS, INC.
SAN DIEGO, CALIFORNIA
```

"Sounds impressive," Gabe said. "What the hell does it mean?"

"I swear to God, Gabe, this shit is better than sex. Here, let me show you." He plugged an outlet box into a yellow extension cord, turned on one of the computers, and typed in a quick sequence of commands. After a few seconds the screen lit up in a colorful burst of animated graphics:

```
WELCOME TO HIPPOCRATES. PLEASE ENTER PATIENT I.D.
   NUMBER, AGE, SEX, AND CHIEF COMPLAINT.
```

"There you go," Jefferson said. "Sit down. You've got to try it."

"Look, Michael. Why don't you just tell me—"

"No, no, no, no, no. You got to see it for yourself.

This is the world's greatest diagnostic software program. You will not *believe* this baby." He set up a folding chair and pushed Gabe into it. "Go ahead," he said. "Give it a case."

"What do you mean?"

"You know. A real patient. Or make one up if you want."

"Michael, come on. I don't want to play computers. I wanted to have a drink and hear about your life. It's been a couple of years."

"Gabe, baby, this *is* my life. My love, my wife. Come on, just one quick case. Fifteen minutes. As a personal favor. If it fails to amaze, I buy."

Gabe sighed. It was going to be computers or nothing. "All right, all right," he said, smiling ruefully at his friend's enthusiasm. "So what is this stupid thing supposed to do, anyway?"

He typed in Lindsey's name, then answered the questions he was asked. The program was thorough and unimaginative. It followed the same sequence a knowledgeable clinician might, except that it skipped nothing. Within a few minutes Gabe was back in the ER, reliving the previous Monday morning.

The machine led him through a process that corresponded very closely to the things he and Watkins had actually done, up to the point where they had ordered the third dose of Hyperstat. It then recommended:

SEND SERUM FOR MAO INHIBITOR ACTIVITY.

Gabe looked up from the screen. "I sent out a postmortem sample. We don't have the results yet."

"No problem," Jefferson said. "Just hit NA—Not Available."

By the end of forty-five minutes the machine had

asked several hundred questions. It asked him please to wait, then provided the following:

PROVISIONAL DIAGNOSIS: LINDSEY TROUTMAN

●1. HYPERTENSIVE CRISIS SECONDARY TO MONOAMINE OXIDASE INHIBITOR REACTION. (PROBABILITY = 0.74)

●2. MALIGNANT HYPERTENSION SECONDARY TO RENAL NECROSIS (PROBABILITY = 0.08)

●3. PHEOCHROMACYTOMA (PROBABILITY = 0.06)

CAUSE OF DEATH

●1. CVA SECONDARY TO TOXIC REACTION (PROBABILITY = 0.87)

●2. CVA SECONDARY TO CONGENITAL ABNORMALITY (PROBABILITY = 0.11)

●3. CVA SECONDARY TO CEREBRAL TRAUMA (PROBABILITY = 0.02)

RECOMMENDATION

CONSULT MAINFRAME FILES FOR CROSSMATCH.

"Hmmmm." Michael was looking over his shoulder. "Interesting. Real case?"

"Yeah." Gabe said. "And I'm really hot to find what it was that killed her. Right away."

"Give me a few hours," Jefferson said. "Once I get everything hooked up I'll patch back into the UC–San Diego mainframe and see what they've got."

"What are you talking about?"

"That's the beauty of this thing." Jefferson patted the computer cabinet fondly. "Medicine is not just a standard set of fixed illnesses anymore. Since we got computers to help us look, we're finding all kinds of new patterns of disease that don't fit the standard patterns. With this baby, you get a case you're not sure of, you can compare it to the two-hundred twenty thousand patient records in the UCSD mainframe. It does a first-approximation match using any five key criteria you pick. Like maybe for this patient we have high blood pressure, sudden onset, no response to meds, bleeders in the retina, and normal white count. It'll spit out any other cases that match that clinical picture."

"And you can do that from here?"

"Sure. Once I get all set up. I can't get full text of the charts, though. You'd have to go down to San Diego for that."

Gabe whistled. "Not bad, Professor. Not bad at all."

Jefferson shrugged modestly. "I've got three other seed-money partners in the company so far," he said in an overly casual voice. "We're going for a second round of private financing later this year. We hope to take the whole thing public in about eighteen months. I could maybe cut you in for some second-round placement if you're really . . ."

Gabe felt a hand on his arm. It was Kate. She wore a tan trench coat thrown over her shoulders. Under the coat she was wearing a charcoal-gray cocktail dress with a string of small pearls, a single matching pearl in each ear. Her hair was still damp from the shower. She gave him a kiss on the cheek and held out her hand to Michael. She then linked her arm in Gabe's, and listened politely while Jefferson went on about his software company.

Gabe was touched by her easy familiarity. It was if they had stepped back into their old life together. He knew that Kate had little interest in medical software. But she could not have been more gracious.

"So listen, you guys," she said at last. "Hold on a second. It's coming up to dinnertime. And I'm starving. Michael? Would you care to join us?"

"I don't know." Michael shook his head. "I guess not. I got a lot more setting up to do."

"Listen, Michael," Gabe said. "I'd like to hear what you find. Let's get together for breakfast."

"Sure thing," Jefferson said. "Nutrition rounds at seven sharp in the hotel coffeeshop?"

"You're on," Gabe said. "I'll see you there." As they were turning to leave, Jefferson caught Kate's arm. "Hey, Katie," he said. "I almost forgot. That big race you got coming up next week?"

"Uh-huh?"

Jefferson stuck out his lower lip, lowered his eyelids, and nodded twice. "I've seen that kick of yours on TV, girl. I think you're going to smoke 'em."

She beamed. "Well thank you, Michael. I'll try."

"You look very elegant tonight," Gabe said as they crossed the exhibit hall. He tried to put his arm around her waist, but she slipped away, shaking her head.

"Look. Gabe. I feel that way too. But I get a little nervous when we're around these Kimberley people. I still feel pretty shaky in this job. So cool it a little, okay?"

"Hey. Sure. I'll be on my best behavior."

She gave him a worried look. "You really think you can stand it?" she asked. "Hanging out all evening with a bunch of boring drug-company types?"

"With you, darling, anything."

"You won't even *be* with me, most likely," she said, shaking her head in resignation. "These people are a trip. They'll probably have the seating all arranged."

11

Kimberley Labs had four exhibit spaces next to the main entrance of the exhibit hall. A small army of blue-blazered young men and women swarmed over the site like worker bees, setting out a variety of freebies—note pads, refrigerator magnets, four-color pens, T-shirts, and coffee mugs—each with the Kimberley logo.

Sheila Sparks, Kimberley's public relations director, stood on a platform in back, talking into a cellular telephone. She was a tall, blond woman with a small, pale face. She was wearing a white linen suit with padded shoulders. Her long dangling earrings and straight blond shoulder-length hair made her look like a priestess in some obscure religious ceremony, one in which she would be worshiped, baptized, or sacrificed.

Gabe had forgotten about Sheila. Of course she would be here. Coordinating publicity and company exhibits was her job.

"Sheila!" Kate called, holding up a hand to catch her attention.

Sheila looked around, saw them, smiled, and held up a long white finger.

Kate gestured in her direction. "That's Sheila

Sparks," Kate said. "She's our VP of public relations." They watched as Sheila spoke into the phone and shook her head, pivoting on one high heel, twisting a strand of hair around her finger.

Gabe nodded, licking his lips. "She wants me to do a column on Kimberley's new antiherpes drug. I've been resisting."

"Virazine. Yes." Kate nodded, smiling. "Sheila's a hard worker. You have to give her that. She uses her looks and plays up to men a little too much for my taste, but she's incredibly good at what she does. She's quite lovely, isn't she?" Unlike many women he'd known, Kate did not automatically consider an attractive woman a personal threat.

Sheila, still on the phone, glanced back at them across a display of Kimberley golf balls. Gabe felt the tremor of recognition in her deep-set green eyes. She turned away quickly, cupping the telephone receiver with her shoulder.

Kate took his arm and stood on tiptoe to whisper in his ear, "She's one of my few women friends at the company. I know you don't particularly care for what she's doing, but do try to be nice, won't you?"

"I'm always nice," he said, looking down at the rows of red and white coffee mugs. An injured fly had fallen into one of them. It was lying on its back, banging its wings helplessly against the sides of the cup.

Gabe had met Sheila at the Kimberley hospitality suite at the Seattle Westin at a medical meeting several months before. Her odd, astringent beauty and her bright banner of long blond hair made every man—and woman—in the room intensely aware of her presence. He had been taken by her attentive, slightly disordered manner, her air of brainy vulnerability.

He had come to her full of righteous outrage over a recent scandal: Kimberley had provided the FDA with faked evidence of the effectiveness of Standine, a new arthritis drug. Sheila had been fully sympathetic to his concerns and was able to provide answers for all his questions: the company had been victimized by an unscrupulous research facility. She assured him that Kimberley staffers had been completely unaware of the deception. Ed Elias had pledged to redo the testing under rigorous FDA supervision.

The evening the conference closed, Sheila had invited him to join her for dinner at a combination restaurant and bookstore in Seattle's university district. It was raining heavily and by the time they arrived their clothes were soaked through.

They huddled together in a corner booth next to the fireplace. They ate oysters and salmon and drank too much champagne and she told him about her life. She had worked with Dean Storch at Crystal Labs and had followed him west a few months earlier. She was lonely and friendless and had been throwing herself into her work. They talked until their clothes had dried. Against his better judgment, Gabe accepted her invitation to go to her suite for a nightcap.

She had left him waiting in the living room for nearly twenty minutes. When she finally emerged from the bedroom she was wearing a sheer black-silk robe. She sat close to him on the couch, looking out over the lights of the city. They talked of this and that. At last she put down her glass, gave him a long, lingering kiss on the mouth, and brought her lips close to his ear.

"I want you to fuck me," she said.

Gabe had tried to put it as nicely as he could. But

77

once Sheila saw that he meant to refuse, the flood-gates of embarrassment and anger broke open. Some-how, in the process of kindness and lies that he had called up in his effort to spare her feelings, he found himself unwittingly offering himself to Sheila in an even more surprising way: as a friend.

"Be nice to her, Gabe," Kate was saying. "She's an odd duck, I know. I was put off a little, too, at first. But when you get to know her you find that she's really quite vulnerable and innocent inside."

Sheila had disappeared behind a blue velvet screen that served as the backdrop for the Kimberley booth. Heads turned as she came out to meet them. She wore a black cape slung over her shoulders.

"Sorry," she said, giving Kate a quick peck on the cheek. "We've been having some problems with the union. Hello, Dr. Austin." She extended a pale white hand. "How nice to see you again." She seemed to be looking at the center of his chest. Her cheeks were flushed like those of a woman run-ning a fever.

"Sheila's been one of my best friends at the com-pany," Kate said. "I'm such a dummy in the busi-ness world. She's been teaching me a lot about how things work in the corporate culture."

"That's not true at all," Sheila said, pleased by Kate's praise. "She is *such* a natural." She turned to Gabe. "She's good. She really is."

They met a group of other Kimberley people in the hotel lobby and were soon on their way across town with a party of thirty-five. Sheila had evidently ar-ranged the whole thing, and when they arrived the restaurant manager was waiting to discuss a number of last-minute details with her. A smiling PR aide directed them to their seats.

Kate had been placed near the head of the table

with a row of Kimberley executives. Gabe found himself on a narrow upholstered bench against the wall at the far end of the table with a group of junior sales reps and a recently retired marketing executive. He was not altogether surprised to find himself sitting next to Sheila.

12

The private dining room was hot and crowded. The waiters kept bringing in latecomers, squeezing them in until Sheila's earrings brushed the shoulder of Gabe's jacket. He was intensely aware of her understated perfume. She had put on tortoiseshell half-glasses to read the menu.

He saw that she was a great favorite with the sales reps. One after another came up to speak to her on some pretext, then stayed around to flirt. It was incredible to see the way she massaged their egos while keeping them at arm's length. The restaurant manager came to check with her on three separate occasions. He seemed determined to make sure the food and service were completely to her liking.

They were interrupted by the wine steward, a distinguished older man in a white vest who wore the silver chain of his office with a quiet dignity. After some discussion, Sheila ordered wine for the table. After the steward went away, Sheila brought her lips close to Gabe's ear.

"You *can* still talk to me, you know," she said, her face aglow. "I won't bite." She pulled at her gold necklace with both hands, as if she were attempting to hold herself on a short leash. "Go ahead," she said. "Ask me how I'm doing." She sipped at her wine, smiling over her shoulder at him. Despite the soft light, her pupils were fully expanded. Only a thin rim of green iris remained.

"So, Sheila." Gabe smiled ruefully. "How *are* you doing?" She had removed her glasses. It made her look more girlish and ethereal.

Sheila glanced at the portly gentleman on her right. He had taken off his hearing aid and was poking at it with his salad fork. "I'm not really hard of hearing," he was explaining to someone across the table. "It's just the high frequencies I have trouble with."

"Pretty miserable, if you really want to know," Sheila said, sipping from her glass. "Running around like a madwoman all day. Lonely and crazy at night. I took your advice. I went to an AA meeting."

"Yeah?" He glanced across at her half-empty wineglass. "How was it?"

"Interesting. Kind of depressing." She made a disgusted face. "I sat around for a couple of hours, yakking and smoking. They were very nice to me. But they were all so old." She raised her wineglass in an ironic toast. "Here's to them. Long may they wave."

"It was brave of you to go," Gabe said.

She shook her head in grim resignation. "I don't think I'm ready to stop drinking yet. I suppose I'm going to get drunk and bore you to tears again." She smiled dazzlingly across the table at an admirer.

"You don't bore me, Sheila," Gabe said.

"No?" She smiled beguilingly, sticking out her lower lip. "You don't think I'm hopeless, then?"

Gabe shook his head. "I think someone hurt you very badly somewhere back in your past. You've been trying to deal with it by working and drinking and sex and drugs."

The blood rushed to her face. She looked across at him through the eyes of a tormented, anguished little girl. "Who . . . who have you been talking to?" she said.

"No one," he said. "Just a guess. You remind me of somebody."

"Who?"

"Lois," he said. "Her name was Lois."

Lois Williams had been a patient of Gabe's during his fourth-year psychiatry clerkship. She was beautiful, she was twenty-three, and she had seduced several of her male doctors. The chief resident explained that Lois had been sexually abused by her father. "You've got to make me one promise," the chief resident had said as he finished presenting her case. "Don't fuck her."

Gabe was outraged. "Of course I won't fuck her!"

"Don't be too sure," the chief resident had said. "She's seductive as hell. She wants you to. It would be pretty understandable if you did. A lot of other doctors have."

"Well, I won't," Gabe had insisted. "I'm not that kind of guy."

He had seen Lois daily for the six weeks of his clerkship. At first, she had been deeply depressed. But as Gabe continued to meet with her, she gradually became more animated. She explained how powerless and guilty she had felt when her father forced his attentions on her. She had repeatedly asked Gabe if he found her attractive. She blushed becomingly and was suitably embarrassed when she described her fantasies of making love with him. She curled up in her chair, giving him well-timed flashes of her black underwear. Toward the end she had stopped wearing underwear.

Gabe had kept his promise. It had not been easy. He had felt himself approaching the danger zone on several occasions, but he had not given in. When they shook hands and said goodbye on the last day of his clerkship, he had every reason to hope that their sessions together had done some good.

His replacement had not been as strong. Lois had seduced him after their third session. Later that evening she had checked herself out of the hospital against medical advice and had jumped off the Golden Gate Bridge.

Sheila had become involved in a conversation with the hearing-aid man. Gabe looked across at her profile—the short, perfect nose, the long line of her jaw. It wasn't her looks that reminded him of Lois. It was her deep conviction that she was of little or no value, that in spite of her great talent and many accomplishments she could be nothing without a man.

Gabe looked down the table. A knot of interested listeners had formed around Kate. There were several people standing behind her chair, waiting to talk to her. Sheila tugged at his arm.

"Your friend Kate has become quite a celebrity," she said. "She's got it all, doesn't she?" She turned to face him. "Money. Fame. Success on the women's marathon circuit. She's certainly got *you* in her hip pocket." She shook her head in resignation. "She's about to be famous too. I've been grooming her for the Virazine media tour."

"What tour is that?"

"If she wins the marathon next week, she's going

out to promote our new antiherpes drug. It's a new public relations thing. You know, the talk shows, the whole . . ."

There was a ripple of conversation, a turning of heads. Sheila looked behind them, bringing a finger to her lips.

"What is it?" Gabe asked.

"Oh, Jesus. The top brass. That's all I need." Sheila rose from her seat, flashing her best professional smile.

Gabe turned his head. A party of eight, all in formal dress, hovered near the door. A short, athletic, white-haired man in a white dinner jacket was walking briskly toward the other end of the table. As everyone watched, he bent down and whispered in Kate's ear. She looked up, smiled, and nodded.

"That must be Elias," Gabe said.

"The little king himself." Sheila smiled wickedly. "You know that he and Kate . . ."

"Yeah," Gabe said, "don't remind me."

"There was a lot of talk about that around the company. The old man recruiting his—" She broke off suddenly, looking behind him with a stiff grimace of a smile. Gabe felt a firm hand on his shoulder.

"Hello there, old man. Long time no see."

It was Dean Storch. His hair had gone gray, his hairline had receded, he was thicker in the waist, and he had traded his glasses for contacts. But he had the same thin, hard mouth and the same bright, ironic blue eyes.

Gabe stood up and they slapped each other on the back. "Hello, Dean. It's great to see you. How the hell are you doing?" He saw that Storch had had his teeth fixed.

"Getting along. Just getting along." Dean seemed oddly restrained, as if his finely tailored dinner jacket and shiny black shoes prevented a more elaborate display of affection. But his eyes twinkled with undisguised pleasure. "Hello, Sheila," he said. "Taking good care of my old student?"

"Yes, sir, Dr. Storch," she said.

"So you're a big-time drug executive now," Gabe said.

"No, not really," Storch said modestly. "Ed is the hero of the piece. I'm just a bit player. I tag along, do the dirty work, and clean up some of the messes." He turned away to shake hands with one of the sales reps.

Gabe looked closely at his old friend. He had abandoned his old go-to-hell manner and become a genial and deferential company insider. Gabe was shocked. He wondered how much Elias was paying him.

"I've been meaning to write you a fan letter," Storch said, coming back to Gabe as if he had not been interrupted. "That column of yours is damn impressive. And I see you on TV all the time. Quite a nice little niche you've carved out for yourself." Storch put a hand on Gabe's shoulder and turned to look up the table. His voice dropped to a whisper. "Have you met Lord Edmund yet?"

"No."

"Well, you simply must. Historic occasion and all. Sheila, you won't mind if I just borrow . . ."

"No, no. Don't let me interrupt your dinner," Elias boomed, hurrying around to their end of the table. He was a youthful man of sixty with a tanned, boyish face. There was nothing boyish about his eyes. He walked up to Gabe, extending a small, hard hand.

"Dr. Austin. A pleasure, sir. I'm a great admirer of yours, young man. Oh, I know we've crossed swords now and then." He waved it all away. "But

I want you to know you have some real friends here at Kimberley. Some real friends indeed."

"Mr. Elias, if you can get people like Dean and Sheila and Kate to work with you, you have my full attention and respect."

"Call me Ed," Elias said, his eyes twinkling. "Funny you should mention that. We've been talking about adding your name to that list. We very much appreciated that second column on Standine. You made an honest mistake and you admitted it. You don't know how rare that is in journalism these days. You must come up and visit our new headquarters. Do you play squash by any chance?"

"I used to play a little back in medical school."

"Excellent. You simply *must* drop up and see us. Bring your squash things. We'll have a little game." He put his hand on Gabe's arm. "Have Kate or Sheila set it up for you. Hello, Robert. How are you? How's that pretty wife of yours?" He reached past Gabe's elbow to shake a proffered hand.

The procession swept on. Dean left Gabe with his card and a promise to call. After they left, everyone at the table let out a deep breath.

"So that's Ed Elias."

"That's him," Sheila said. "What do you think?"

"Pretty impressive," Gabe said. "Where does Dean fit into the picture?"

"He's our executive VP now. A very big cheese. The heir apparent, some people say."

"Sounds like you don't much care for him."

"Dean? Oh, no. He's . . . he's all right. He's just . . . well, let's just say he loses his polished manners and his posh British accent sometimes."

A young sales rep with a guardsman mustache leaned in between Gabe and Sheila and tried to get her to go somewhere with him after dinner. While they were talking, Kate came by.

"Bad news, Gabe." She stood behind him, her hands on his shoulders. "We've run into a major problem at the company. Ed has asked me to sit in on an emergency strategy meeting." She made a wry face. "It looks like we're going to be running pretty late. I'm afraid I'll have to take a rain check for the evening. Maybe Sheila could take you out gambling."

"I'd be delighted," Sheila said.

"Sure," Gabe said. "No problem."

"Sorry." Kate smiled. "We'll find something fun to do tomorrow night. Don't you guys lose all your money now." She squeezed Gabe's shoulder, shrugged, and made her way back to her seat.

It was just after 1:00 A.M. when the cab dropped Gabe back at the Hilton. He ran the gauntlet of the first-floor casino, took the elevator to the top floor, and knocked on Kate's door. There was no answer for a long time. He was about to give up when he sensed an eye at the peek hole. A moment later, Kate opened the door.

"Sorry, sweetie. We're still working." She stepped out into the hall. Gabe caught a glimpse of Storch, Elias, and several other Kimberley executives on the leather couches in their shirt sleeves, a thick stack of files and computer printouts on the coffee table before them.

"So what's up?" he asked.

"Some stupid business emergency. Jesus. Am I tired." She pulled the door nearly closed behind her and raised herself on tiptoe to kiss him on the lips. She leaned heavily against him, pressing her temple against his chest. Her hair smelled of cigarettes.

"No parties for this girl tonight, I'm afraid," she

said. She looked up at him with tired eyes. "I guess you should probably stay downstairs. Sorry to stand you up like this. The bullshit we do go through, huh?" She straightened his tie and brushed a piece of lint from his lapel. "Did you and Sheila have a good time?"

"Just dandy," he said. "I won twenty dollars at blackjack. She lost about a hundred on the slots."

"That sounds about par for the course. Should I be jealous?"

He shook his head. "She's a little too neurotic for me."

"Good. I'm too tired to be jealous." She put a hand on the door.

"What kind of an emergency?" he said.

She took his arm and moved a step away from the door. "There's been a big run-up in Kimberley's stock price. There's a rumor that somebody's about to attempt a hostile takeover." She gestured back over her shoulder. "These poor guys don't have a clue what the hell's happening. Ed's livid. We're trying to calm him down. Don't tell anybody, okay?"

"My lips are sealed." He slipped his arms around her. "I miss you," he said.

She nodded. "This is a real test, isn't it? Maybe if we can make it through this weekend . . . Tomorrow night, okay?"

"Sure."

"Really," she said. "Tomorrow. Don't forget." She gave him a sisterly kiss, then darted her tongue into the corner of his mouth.

13

The phone woke Gabe early the next morning. It was still dark outside. He could see the neon signs flickering outside his window.

"Hey, Gabe. Michael Jefferson. Rise and shine, baby. Got something hot for you."

"Michael." Gabe sat up. "What time is it?"

"Five-thirty. I decided to let you sleep in. I've been up running your case match most of the night."

Gabe came instantly awake. "Yeah? What'd you find?"

"San Diego has two cases with a full five-point match on a first-run approximation. But I can't get you the full medical record online. I called Florence—you remember, my administrative assistant. She's going to pull the records for you first thing this morning. It's mildly illegal, so you'll have to get there before she goes home at noon. Southwest Air has a one-stop at seven-ten. I went ahead and got you a seat. You can pick up your ticket at the airport. You need to be at the front door of the hotel in forty minutes. The shuttle driver will be waiting. He's been exorbitantly tipped. I knew you'd want to hop on this right away."

Gabe showered, dressed, packed, and slipped a hurriedly written note under Kate's door. At seven-fifteen he was in the air. At ten-fifteen he was walking into the emergency department at UCSD.

The nursing station was full of the smell of fresh coffee. The sun was shining in through the windows of the empty waiting room, and there was not an ambulance to be seen. A tall black resident in a crisp white skirt looked up from her *Los Angeles Times* and directed him to Florence Lehman's office. As he neared the door Gabe heard her talking on the phone.

". . . and I'm telling you all IV tubes are not the same, Mr. Purvis. Yes. We've given your brand a good try. They have a defect rate of about one in a hundred. *Defects,* Mr. Purvis. Air leaks, Mr. Purvis. Air *embolisms,* Mr. Purvis." She looked up at Gabe, waved, and held up a finger. She was a thin, nervous woman with a long, thin nose and bright, birdlike eyes. A yellow pencil was tucked under the earpiece of her rimless glasses.

"Have you ever seen an air embolism, Mr. Purvis? It can stop your heart like flipping a switch. I'm asking you, Mr. Purvis, would you want your own *mother* to get an IV with defective tubing? Well, I'm sorry she's dead, but you get the idea. Yes, I'll tell him you said so. You too. Have a nice day." She put down the phone, made a check next to an item on a long list, and shook her head. "Stupid people," she said, coming around the desk to shake Gabe's hand. "I just don't have a lot of patience with stupid people anymore."

"You never did, Florence."

"Smart and funny is best. Smart and dull is not so bad." She made a thumb-over-the-shoulder gesture in the direction of Michael's office. "But dumb and boring . . ." She made a large *X* in the air over the telephone. "So. Dr. Austin. I'm so glad you two are working together again." She lowered her voice. "You're the only one that can get him interested in anything besides that silly computer program of his."

She led him into a big, attractive office with high windows and an electronics bench running the length of one wall. Like many academic researchers with entrepreneurial tendencies, Jefferson ran his fledgling company out of his university office. Florence served as both unofficial ER director and chief corporate administrator, yet was so efficient that she was able to go home at noon every day. She closed the door and waved Gabe toward the executive chair behind the big walnut desk.

"So how's the boy wonder doing?" he asked, settling into the deep leather cushions.

"Dr. Jefferson? Same as ever. Convinced he's going to get rich with this new program of his."

"Is he?"

"Not a chance." She extended her lower lip and shook her head.

"What's the matter? It doesn't work?"

"It works fine. There are just two problems: He doesn't know a thing about marketing. And I don't think you docs are about to give up your magic powers to some stupid machine." She shrugged. "I could be wrong. Now let me just make sure you have everything you need: the two charts you wanted, sharpened pencils, yellow pads, a phone. I'll get you a fresh cup of coffee. Lots of milk, no sugar, right?"

By five that evening Gabe had read each chart three times. He had called all the key doctors and nurses who had taken care of both patients and had made appointments to see the next of kin of each of the deceased patients that evening. As he passed through the ER, he saw the tall black resident again.

She had blood on her coat, vomit on her shoes, and a glazed, vacant look in her eye.

Half an hour later he was driving his rental car past the junkyards and the defunct gas stations of an industrial-residential district in southeast San Diego. He consulted the yellow pad on the seat beside him, then pulled up in front of a small frame house with chipped green siding. The bushes in the yard were untrimmed, as if to screen the cracked windows from view. The faint ocean breeze carried the smell of a nearby oil refinery.

The driveway and garage were empty. The porch sagged under his step. No one answered his knock.

He returned to the car, tuned in to the local NPR station, and listened to an interview with an accused serial murderer. The reporter asked the man why he had killed all those people. The accused killer replied that killing people was just like anything else. After the first few times, the whole business became routine—no more outlandish than brushing your teeth or eating your breakfast.

It was a little after six-thirty when a dented brown Toyota turned into the driveway. A pretty Chicano woman got out. She carried a plump two-year-old girl in one arm, a bag of groceries in the other. Gabe came up behind her while she was struggling with her keys.

"*Buenas tardes. Señora Rodriguez?*" The little girl squirmed to be let down.

"*Sí?*" She looked back at Gabe, irritation and suspicion on her face.

"*Dr. Gabe Austin de la Hospital Universidad para servirle. Soy quien llame por telefono en la tarde. Puedo avudarle con su bolsa?*"

She appeared mildly amused by Gabe's accent. She

let the little girl slip down her leg to the porch. "You can speak English," she said. "Come on, *corazon.* Inside." She pushed the child inside and stood blocking the doorway, holding the bag of groceries like a shield.

"Why do you want to know about Juan?"

"We're trying to find what made him so ill."

"Trying to find out? The doctor said he had a bad blood vessel in his brain. He said Juan was born that way, that it could have happened at any time."

"That may be. But we've had two very similar deaths. I'm trying to find out what they might have in common."

She considered. Gabe was glad he had worn his suit. He did his best to look trustworthy and responsible. "Well," she said at last. "Come in, then."

The overhead light sent two large cockroaches scuttling for cover. The girl clung to her mother's leg, looking up suspiciously at Gabe. Mrs. Rodriguez put the bag of groceries on a rickety kitchen table.

"Carmelita, this is one of the doctors who took care of Juan at the hospital. Can you say hello?" The child bit at her knuckle, looking up at Gabe blankly.

"Mama? When is Juan coming home?"

"He's not coming back anymore, *mi vida,*" she said in a dead, level voice. "Juan's died and gone to heaven, like I told you."

"But when is he coming *home?* You said you'd read us a story."

"I'll read you a story after supper. Now you run along and play with your doll."

The girl made a face and tried to hide behind her mother's skirt.

"I said you run along now. *Andale.*"

The girl left the room in a pout, dragging her feet. Gabe followed Mrs. Rodriguez into the small kitchen.

"Coffee?" She waved him to a chair.

"Yes, thank you." She made two cups of instant coffee with hot water from the tap. Gabe forced himself to take a small sip. He opened his folder on the kitchen table.

"Perhaps we could start back before Juan was born. Were there any problems with the pregnancy?"

Gabe asked questions for the better part of an hour. Mrs. Rodriguez answered briefly, clearly, and without emotion. She said little about herself and volunteered no information on her own. At one point the girl came back carrying her doll and sat in her mother's lap.

There was no history of depression or high blood pressure or eating disorders. By the time he ran out of questions, Gabe knew that Juan had been a normal, healthy boy. He'd had all the normal childhood diseases—ear infections, occasional asthma, cold sores, strep throat, measles. Nothing out of the ordinary. He had attended an excellent school run as a demonstration project by the university and received top-rate medical care. Mrs. Rodriguez had a complete copy of his outpatient medical record.

Juan's father had had tuberculosis at one time. Mrs. Rodriguez had not seen him for nearly two years.

"Do you have a picture of Juan I could have?"

She brought him a framed school photo of a shy, dark-haired boy with one front tooth missing. There was a formal, serious look about him, as if he realized he had become the man of the house.

"He looks like a nice kid."

"He was a bright boy," she said. "A good boy." There was no trace of emotion in her voice.

"Your English is excellent," he said. "You must have spoken it as a child."

She shook her head, smiling for the first time. "No. I have worked very hard to be an American."

"You're being very brave about all this."

She looked across at him calmly. "He is happy in heaven with the angels," she said. "I have this one to take care of now." She took his cup, carried it to the sink, and washed it vigorously with a red plastic brush. "I was crazy at first. *Muy loca.* They took me to see the priest. I had not been to Mass since I can't remember when, but the priest said it didn't matter. Jesus is always there. I have to make dinner for my daughter now. Do you have any more questions?"

14

Robert Blumberg's widow lived in a big multilevel redwood house on the top of a hill overlooking the San Diego harbor. Gabe drove up a well-lighted driveway between rows of young trees propped up by sturdy green stakes. He parked beside a white Mercedes station wagon and walked up a wide flight of brightly lit steps to a spacious deck. He rang the bell, waited, and rang again.

There was a narrow pane of glass beside the door. A short, round-faced woman was coming slowly down the steps. She wore a cranberry polo shirt and baggy white painter's pants. She stood for a moment before opening the door, unaware of his gaze, a finger of her left hand touching her lower lip, as if she were listening to some distant music. It was several seconds before she answered the door.

"You must be Dr. Austin. I'm Amy Blumberg." Her white, crooked teeth stood out in her deeply tanned face. The hand she gave him was large and capable.

"I'm sorry about your husband," Gabe said.

She nodded absently. "Come in," she said. "I was just getting the children settled." She seemed to be speaking to him from a great distance, relying on a life-long habit of conviviality to keep things moving along.

It was the kind of house you get when a good architect pulls out all the stops—skylights, courtyards, white vaulted ceilings. Gabe felt as though he'd walked into one of those four-dollar architecture magazines. A dozen vases of fading flowers stood on a long rosewood dining table. As they passed a long hallway he could hear children's voices.

"Would you like a cup of tea?"

"That would be nice."

He followed her to a large, open kitchen. She opened a rosewood cabinet above the butcher block counter.

"Is Earl Grey all right? We do have some others."

"Earl Grey will be fine."

She poured cold water into a teapot, added two tea bags, put it into the microwave, and leaned back against the counter. "So what exactly is it you wanted to know about Robert?"

"His medical history. Everything that happened during the last few days before he went to the hospital."

Her eyes blurred and she looked down at the terracotta tiles of the kitchen floor. "I don't understand," she said at last. "I would think they'd have all that in his hospital chart."

"I'm looking for things that might not be in the chart."

"You don't think . . . there was some kind of a mistake?"

Gabe shook his head. "No. He had the best care possible. They . . ."

The microwave beeped. She took out the pot and put it on a tray. "Let's go into the living room," she said.

She led him back through the house to a large room with couches and a stone fireplace, waving him to a seat on a long white lamb's-wool sofa that looked out over the harbor. She moved a straw knitting basket and sat down on the matching love seat at his right.

"Let me make sure I understand," she said. "What exactly was it that Robert had?"

"He had very high blood pressure that didn't respond to medication," Gabe said. He could see the moon reflected in the black water of the lap pool on the patio, a bright, glowing sphere that looked as if it had been sliced in half with a knife.

"They called it something that made it sound like cancer," she said. "I was going to go back and ask. But I never did."

Gabe nodded. "Malignant hypertension. That's the official name for it. I see how it could be misleading."

"But it doesn't have anything to do with cancer?"

"No. Your husband did not have cancer."

"I didn't think so." A large painting dominated the wall across from him: A man in a shirt and tie was sitting on the side of a bed, pulling at his shoes. A nude woman lay half-covered, looking away from him. It was warm and loosely painted and full of soft flecks of color. Gabe wondered if the woman might be Amy herself.

"I'm sorry I'm so confused," she said. "It . . . it feels like a bomb has been dropped on my life." A single tear ran down her cheek. She wiped it away with a white lace handkerchief.

"It was a very unusual clinical picture," Gabe said. "I'm here because we've seen this same pattern in several other people. I'm trying to find out what they might have had in common."

She stood up suddenly. "It's so stuffy in here. Perhaps—if it's not too cold for you—we could take our tea out onto the patio?"

He carried the tea tray to a glass-topped table between two lounge chairs next to the pool. The breeze from the ocean had turned cool. She warmed up his tea, then went inside for a sweater, bringing him back a long sheepskin coat that smelled of wood smoke and the ocean.

"I'll bet you used to sit out here with your husband in the evenings," Gabe said.

"Yes." She nodded, smiling at the memory. "Even before we built the house we used to come up here with our tea in a Thermos bottle."

"Your husband designed the house?"

She nodded. "We chose the paintings first. I have a small gallery downtown. He designed the house around them."

"It's lovely."

She nodded. "It is, isn't it? It's so odd the way things work out. We'd been planning it for more than eight years, choosing the site, saving up the money, revising the plans, getting all the permits they require these days." She rolled her eyes at the dark sky. "We finally finished it last spring. And then Robert died. There's probably some kind of moral in that, don't you think?'' She poured herself another cup of tea.

"What will you do?"

She sipped at the steaming cup. "I haven't decided yet. I suppose I'll look for a cheaper house nearby. The kids are in a good school. I'd hate to have to move them, but I can't afford to stay. Even if I could, there would be too many memories.'' She let out a long sigh. "Robert was always in such perfect health. He ran, he played tennis, he used the exercise machines at his health club."

"He had no medical problems that you knew of?"

"Oh, his back bothered him sometimes. All architects have bad backs. He had a bunion taken off a couple of years ago and some moles removed before that.''

"Did he ever take any medications for depression or high blood pressure?"

"No.''

"Eating disorders?"

"No.''

"Nothing else?"

"Nothing very impressive. He had a funny rash on his back a month or so ago. It had an unusual name. Something about roofs.''

"Shingles?"

"Yes, that's it. It hurt him horribly. He couldn't even stand to have the sheets on his skin. A dermatologist friend gave him something for it.''

"Do you know the dermatologist's name?"

She nodded. "Jeremy Rogers. He and Robert were at Dartmouth together.''

"Was he taking any other medications?"

"He took his vitamins every morning. I don't think he was taking anything else. You're welcome to look at our medicine cabinet.''

The Blumbergs' master bathroom had a door of frosted glass that disappeared into the wall. There was a sunken whirlpool tub and a separate shower stall with brass faucets and handles. A pair of French doors led to a private garden with a hot tub and a view of the city.

Gabe made a list of all the drugs in the medicine cabinet: a multivitamin, niacin, vitamin A, vitamin C, cod liver oil, calcium, Pepto-Bismol, Tylenol No. 3, Medipren, and half a dozen bottles of old prescription drugs. She stood watching quietly while he recorded the names in his pocket notebook.

"The painkillers were for his back?"

"Yes. I sometimes use the Medipren for menstrual cramps."

"The calcium is for you?"

"Yes. Would you like to see the back garden?"

"Sure."

She opened the French doors. They stepped out onto the deck and stood looking out across the steaming hot tub at the lights of the city.

"Sorry to have to make you go through this," he said.

She smiled and shook her head. "Don't be. It's good to talk to someone about it. I never dreamed that Robert might die so young." She shook her head. "For the first time in years I feel completely, totally lost." She put her hands in the pockets of her sweater and took a step away, her back to him, looking up at the sky.

"Everybody wants to give you a little pat and get on with their busy lives," she said. "And you have to let them do that. That's the part that no one understands, even your closest friends." She bent down to pick a fallen branch off the deck. "They send you flowers and covered dishes and they're all so uncomfortable that you have to take care of *them*. After a while I suppose it all closes over and the feeling goes away."

"Never completely, though," Gabe said.

She nodded. "I think so much of Robert these days. More than I ever did when he was alive. I can imagine him sitting, reading the paper in the next room. I can hear his voice. I can even hear him snoring at night." She laughed, shaking her head again. "It's a kind of life after death, I suppose. Well. Enough of that." She turned to face him, her eyes glistening in the lights from the house. "You didn't come up here to hear about my personal problems. Did you find what you were looking for?"

Gabe drove back to the airport, turned in his rental car, and called Kate at her Reno hotel room.

"I got your note," she said. "What did you find?" Her voice seemed strangely distant and reserved. She had presented a slide show on corporate wellness programs at the medical meeting that afternoon. Gabe wondered if she was angry that he'd missed it.

"Two new cases, both of them very similar to Lindsey's. It's a little frightening," he said. "Look, I'm sorry I missed your talk. How did it go?"

She let out a long sigh. "Fine. It was very well received. I was really sad you weren't there to hear it. I guess . . . I guess I wanted you to see that I've found a little bit of success in medicine after all."

"Oh, baby. I know you have. Listen. You're famous for your work in setting up wellness programs."

"Next time," she said.

"For sure," he said. "How's your problem at the company working out?"

"It's still pretty complicated," she said. "I can't

talk about it on the phone. I'd love to tell you to come back and we'd have a wild night on the town, but I'll probably have to meet with the executive committee again tonight."

There was a long silence.

"This weekend isn't working out as we'd hoped, is it?" she said at last.

"No. It's not. Sorry I had to run off like this."

"You're forgiven," she said. "I'm sorry I've been such a party-pooper. Are you going back to San Francisco?"

Gabe considered. "If you think you're going to be tied up tonight I probably will," he said. "I need to cross-check Lindsey's history against these two new cases. There're all just too damn much alike. There's got to be something I'm missing."

"Gabe?"

"Yeah?"

"I want to be sure you're going to be able to ride with me in the marathon. Another friend had offered to do it, so I have to let her know."

"Sure. Absolutely."

"Good. It'll really mean a lot to me. Why don't you plan to come over Monday night. I'll pick up some pizza and we can sit in my hot tub and plot our strategy for the race."

15

Alex and Margaret Troutman lived in a stately old Victorian in Bernal Heights. It was perched on the side of a hill three blocks above Mission Street.

Margaret glanced out through a clear spot in the etched-glass window. Her chubby face had a haunted, preoccupied look. She was a shorter, heavier version of her younger sister.

"Gabe! Golly. What a surprise. Alex is at the hospital." She hesitated, pushing her thick glasses up on her nose. She was wearing furry pink slippers and a fuzzy blue running suit.

"Hello, Margaret." He offered her a hug. She was tentative at first. Then she let out a long sigh. Gabe wondered how it was that he got along so much better with the child in this family than he ever had with the parents.

"So how are you doing?" he said.

"Not so good. But come in anyway. You want some coffee?"

"Sure. I have a favor to ask."

The inside of the house had been completely redone, most of it by Margaret herself. There were hardwood floors and oriental carpets, stripped wood trim and white paint. She led him through a cluttered front room into a warm, cozy kitchen that smelled of fresh pastry.

A photo album lay open on the table. She shooed a black cat off a chair and gave Gabe the seat with the view. Margaret sat down across from him, closing the album and pushing it away. "What was it you wanted?" she said.

"I'd like to get a photo of Lindsey."

"Sure. No problem." The cat sulked in a corner, giving him evil looks.

"And I'd like to take a look at her things," he said. "Her room, her purse, the bathroom she used." He looked out across Mission Street and lower Noe Valley. The morning sun shone on the spires of St. Cecilia's and highlighted the wisps of morning fog spilling over the mountain peaks that formed the far side of the valley.

"Her room's a terrible mess," A look of pain and embarrassment crossed Margaret's face. "You're thinking drugs, aren't you?"

"Tell you the truth, I don't know what I'm looking for," he said. "Did she ever say anything to you about a problem with bulimia?"

"Gosh, no. But she always worried about her weight."

"Do you mind if I look in her room?"

Margaret put her face in her hands. "I haven't been able to make myself go up there yet." She bit her bottom lip. "Go ahead. It's upstairs. First door on the right."

"Thanks," Gabe said. He started to get up. "Uh . . . do you smell something burning?"

"Oh, no." She rushed to the oven, opened the door, and let out a cloud of sweet blue-gray smoke. "Darn it anyway," she said. "That's the second time today." She turned on the fan in the hood over the stove, waving ineffectually at the smoke with a hot pad. "I am absolutely coming *apart,* Gabe. Really. Sometimes I think I can hear her up in her room, playing her tapes or talking on the phone. I keep expecting her to come in and ask me about some physics problem or something. Not that I ever knew the least thing about it. I'm such a mathematical moron. I'd just sit there like a dummy while she figured it out for herself. You know what she'd always say?" She threw herself down in her chair, leaning forward on her pudgy arms.

Gabe shook his head.

"She'd say, 'Thanks, Mom.' Like I had really done something. And we'd both laugh. 'Thanks, Mom.' Jesus. What a kid."

Lindsey's room was at the far end of the upstairs hall. A computer-printed sign on the door read:

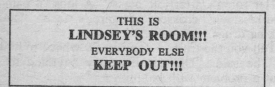

THIS IS
LINDSEY'S ROOM!!!
EVERYBODY ELSE
KEEP OUT!!!

It was a long, dark L-shaped room with a high ceiling. A tall Victorian window looked out at a red brick wall three feet away. Every square inch of the floor was covered by clothes, towels, books, papers, and the other artifacts of the life of a precocious teenage girl. Gabriel had to wade through the debris to get in.

There were books and magazines and cassette tapes and compact discs everywhere. A battery-powered travel alarm was balanced on top of a purple jewelry box on a marble-topped cabinet next to the bed. There was a row of framed cast photos. Many of the books were acting editions of plays. Gabriel spotted copies of *Romeo and Juliet*, *Tom Jones*, and *Murder by Death*.

A red folding travel iron stood on a purple towel that had been spread across the top of a Danish modern student desk. Beside the iron was a thick note pad, its pages cut in the shape of a fat purple pencil. A black trunk next to the desk held a portable CD player and a stack of back issues of *Rolling Stone*, *Vogue*, and *Seventeen*. A dresser with a broken drawer was covered with small bottles and jars of makeup, perfume, and shampoo.

A high canopied bed with wrinkled pink sheets stood at the far end of the room like a safe island in a sea of chaos. A white phone on a long cord was nestled among the sheets. Lindsey had written her name in pink fingernail polish across the back of the receiver. Gabe ran his finger along the raised letters. He felt the stirring of guilt and grief deep inside him.

"Lindsey," he whispered. "I'm sorry. I didn't know what to do to save you. I hope you're at peace. If there was anything I did that hurt you, anything that made things worse, please forgive me."

He heard a knock and turned to see Margaret standing in the doorway, holding a cup and saucer.

"You forgot your coffee," she said. She hovered at the door as if unwilling to come in. "Julia is coming down this weekend," she said. "She has those two young daughters now, so I thought . . . her clothes . . . some of her things . . ." She let out a long, quivering sigh and looked down at the cluttered floor like a bewildered child.

"I'll leave your cup out here in the hall," she said at last. "There's no place to put it."

He found Margaret in the kitchen rolling out a pie crust. She looked up at him apologetically. "I salvaged some of the coffee cake," she said. "It's really not too bad, if you don't mind a little burned sugar. Any luck?" She brought him a large piece of the singed pastry.

"Not really. When's the last time Lindsey stayed home sick from school?"

"You couldn't *make* that girl stay home. She was so darn committed to her theater group. She was so compulsive about never missing even a single rehearsal. It was like the whole drama department depended on her. And I guess they did. How is it?"

He took a bite of the coffee cake. It tasted like a charcoal-broiled sugar doughnut. "Fine," he said.

"They canceled the play she was going to be in. And that wonderful memorial service." She started to cry again. "And they say kids these days have no feelings." She turned away from him and hurried out of the room, her shoulders shaking.

Gabe sat at the table and drank his cold coffee. The cat had recovered its good temper. It crossed the room and began rubbing against his ankles. After a few minutes Margaret came back and sat down across from him. "Oh, God. Sometimes I think I'm never going to stop crying."

"When was the last time she was sick?" he asked.

"It was about two weeks ago. She started feeling really tired. Alex thought she was just staying up too late, but I knew she was really sick. He was on call at the hospital and never seemed to have the time, so I finally took her out to one of the student health doctors at San Francisco State."

"San Francisco State?"

She nodded. "She was taking a Thursday night acting class. A lot of the brighter kids from Lincoln High take college classes in the evening."

"What'd they do for her?"

"The doctor said she had mono. He gave her some pills."

"Pills? For mono?" There is no effective drug treatment for mononucleosis.

"That's right," Margaret said. "Don't ask me what it was. I can never remember drug names. Alex could probably tell you what they were."

16

Gabe drove out to San Francisco State the first thing Monday morning. He found a map of the campus in the massive white cement pyramid that served as the student union. It didn't help. After ten minutes of looking, he still hadn't located the student health center.

He stopped on a little rise to ask a petite Chinese-American girl for directions. She laughed and pointed straight down.

"You're standing on it," she said.

The student health center had been built underground, a long row of plate glass windows set into the side of the little hill. It had been constructed around a light well that contained a tiny Japanese garden. The waiting room was full of very healthy-looking young men and women.

The clinic administrator was a pug-nosed, no-nonsense little woman named Joan DeWitt. She gave him a small, moist hand. "A pleasure, Dr. Austin. I enjoy your columns. We've used some of them as hand-outs. Whoops. Hope that doesn't get me into trouble."

"Feel free," he said. He gave her the note he'd had Margaret write, authorizing the student health center to provide him with a complete copy of Lindsey's medical records. She frowned down at it, tapping a pencil against her chin.

"Of course. I'll have a copy made right away." She picked up her phone. "Marta, could you come in please?" She uncapped a black fountain pen and copied Lindsey's name onto her note pad in small, precise handwriting. "You say this young lady is . . . uh . . . deceased?"

"That's right."

She frowned and shook her head. "That's very rare for us." A willowy African-American woman in jeans and tinted glasses appeared in the doorway.

"Pull this chart for me, will you please?" DeWitt ripped off the page from her note pad and handed it to her.

"Sure thing, Ms. DeWitt."

"How many AIDS deaths have you had here?" Gabe asked.

"Not many." She raised her eyebrows and tapped her pen against the desk. "We get the HIV-positive and the worried well. The more serious cases generally go to more specialized facilities."

Marta returned with a thin chart between heavy manila covers.

"Thank you. Now—let's see what we have." She put on a pair of half-glasses and bent over the open chart. "She was seen by Dr. Carmichael. Dr. Milton Carmichael." She looked up at Gabe, a pained look on her face. "He's a retired military physician. He sees patients here on Mondays and Fridays. Those are our peak days, you see, so I was happy to find a doctor willing to—"

The phone on her desk buzzed. She picked it up, nodded, and glanced at her watch. "Let me just run through this quickly," she said. "We've seen her only once. She came in two weeks ago, complaining of chronic fatigue and sleeping more than usual. She had a slight fever with swollen, tender nodes in her neck. A mono spot test was positive. She was diagnosed as having mononucleosis and received a prescription."

"A prescription for what?" Mono is usually treated with bed rest and plenty of fluids.

"I'm afraid Dr. Carmichael's writing is a little hard to read." She turned the chart around and passed it across the desk. Gabe looked down at the shaky handwriting. It could have been any one of a number of drugs. He became aware of an uneasy feeling in his stomach.

"How can I get ahold of Dr. Carmichael?" he asked.

"I'll have Marta get you his address and phone number. And a copy of the chart. Dr. Carmichael's an avid gardener and he rarely answers his phone during the day. I suggest you go right on out." She stood up. "It's been a pleasure meeting you," she said. "Keep up the good work."

Dr. Carmichael lived on Forty-eighth Street, out near the ocean just north of the zoo. Gabe found the number on one of two identical gates in a high board fence. He made his way along the narrow sidewalk that ran between the front house and a bank of English ivy. It led him to a well-tended dove-gray cottage in back. A rotating sprinkler was soaking the tiny lawn.

No one answered his knock. He followed a trail of

concrete stepping stones past rows of staked raspberry vines around to the back of the cottage.

A slight, wiry man with close-cropped white hair sat at a redwood picnic table, dividing a large pot of ivy into several smaller clay pots. He was wearing a light gray shirt, a red tie, and a blue canvas apron.

"Dr. Carmichael?"

"What? Hello?" He waved Gabe toward him, wiped his hands on a folded towel, and turned up his hearing aid.

"I'm sorry," he said. "The front house is already rented. A nice young couple just out from Illinois. He works for Transamerica. The pyramid people, you know. I'm just potting up some ivy for them to brighten up the place. Wonderful stuff, ivy, if you don't mind baiting for snails and slugs."

"I'm not here about the house."

"What?"

"I said I'm not here about the house." Gabe sat down across the table from him and gave him one of his cards. Carmichael read it slowly, his lips moving.

"Well, Dr. Austin," he said at last. "To what do I owe this pleasure?"

"You saw a patient of mine last week. Lindsey Troutman," Gabe said. He passed his copy of the chart across the table. Carmichael frowned, opened the file folder, and read briefly.

"I'm afraid I don't remember her, Doctor. We see quite a few . . ."

Gabe took the photo of Lindsey out of its envelope and pushed it across to him. Carmichael's weathered face broke into a smile.

"Oh, yes. Of course. Miss Troutman. One of our high school students. A very pleasant young woman." He frowned again. "Is something the matter?"

"Can you tell me what you remember about her?"

Carmichael searched Gabe's face, then frowned down at the table, raising his eyebrows. "Nice girl. Very young. Seventeen going on twenty-seven, if you know what I mean." He squinted his eyes closed. "She had the lead in a school play and was scared to death that she wouldn't be able to perform. Clear symptoms of mononucleosis—sore throat, swollen lymph nodes, a low fever. Half the patients I see out there have it. I did a mono spot test. It was positive."

"How did you treat her?"

"She seemed like a healthy girl and seemed to have a fairly mild case, so I was tempted not to treat her at all. But she seemed so worried that she might have to miss a performance. She really seemed to want me to give her something. I'd just been talking with one of the drug salespeople. A very nice young woman. I can't think of her name. She'd given me a whole drawerful of Virazine—you know, the new antiherpes drug. She was saying that their researchers thought it might turn out to be useful against the whole range of herpes viruses."

Gabe was aware of an intense pounding in his head. "So you figured it might help against mono?" he said.

"Yes. Mono is in the herpes family, of course. And I thought that at the very least it would make her feel more confident about her play. And it had been through all the usual rigorous testing. So it *certainly* wasn't going to do her any harm."

17

I can't believe it," Gabe said, hanging up the phone and looking across the desk at Gertrude. "They were all taking Virazine. Every one of them. What do you know about this stuff?"

Gertrude gave him a concerned look. She dropped her eyes and paused to sip delicately at her tea. "It is hard to believe there could be a problem. The testing for Virazine was done right after the whole Standine scandal. . . ."

"Yeah," Gabe said. "When they were trying to prove that they were purer than pure."

"Yes," Gertrude said. "They were bending over backward to be as thorough and complete as possible. They tested the drug in a much larger number of human volunteers than the regulations require. They even had FDA observers in during the testing. Yes, come in, Jesse. What is it?"

She turned away to answer a question from one of her graduate students. Gabe looked down at his notes. Dr. Carmichael had given Lindsey Troutman Virazine for mono. Jeremy Rogers had given the drug to Robert Blumberg for shingles. And a pediatrician named Howard Metzenbaum at the University School in San Diego had given it to Juan Rodriguez for cold sores.

The student went out, closing the door behind him. Gertrude rolled her chair over to Gabe, a troubled expression on her face.

"These three cases are certainly of great concern," she said. "But you must realize that they do not constitute proof that the high blood pressure that killed these three was a side effect of Virazine."

"I know," he said. "We'll have to gather more cases and get better proof as soon as we can."

"Ed Elias and his friends will not be happy to hear about this. I know they all consider Virazine a very important drug for the future of the company."

"It will not be a real pleasant experience, I'm sure," Gabe said. "So what are you trying to say?"

Gertrude studied him over the rim of her cup. "Perhaps it would be better if I took care of this myself, yes? I do know all the key people out there. Ed Elias. Dean Storch. Arthur McCauley. Even Howard Pearlman, the researcher who developed the drug in the first place. I could send over some copies of the victim's medical records and handle everything by phone. You wouldn't need to be involved."

"No," Gabe said, shaking his head. "I am involved. I'll be seeing Kate tonight. And I hope to see Ed Elias tomorrow."

"You're sure?" Gertrude asked. "I would hate to have something like this become a problem between you and Kate."

Fog had slowed the rush hour traffic on the Golden Gate Bridge to a crawl. Gabe peered out at the brake lights of a white Porsche a yard in front of him. The wipers of his old Volvo station wagon squeaked unmercifully. It took forever to reach the Wolfe Grade

Tunnel. When he came out on the north side, the sun was low in a blue, cloudless sky.

On the radio, a local architect was talking about earthquake-proof housing. In Japan, he explained, the buildings were all built on springs and rubber pads. When the tremors came, the homes and office buildings just jiggled.

Gabe took the San Rafael exit, made a round-the-block detour, and pulled up beside the Federal Express drop box in front of Marin Savings. He let the motor run, looking down at the fat envelope on the seat beside him. It was addressed to Ken Weber, an old fellow student from Gertrude's lab. Ken had gone on to become a highly respected pharmacoepidemiologist. He now worked in the department of post-marketing surveillance for the Food and Drug Administration.

Gabe took a deep breath, got out of the car, dropped the envelope into the box, and took Third Street west to Sir Frances Drake.

The next guest on the talk show was a woman who had written a series of books about vampires. The interviewer asked her if, given the chance, she would herself become a vampire, relinquishing all hope of ever seeing the sun in exchange for eternal life. "Oh, yes," she answered. "Oh my, yes."

Gabe followed Sir Frances Drake west through Kentfield and San Anselmo, all the way to Fairfax. He turned left on Fairfax Avenue, winding his way up into the hills. It was a quiet, green hideaway, far from freeways and cities. Old summer homes stood side by side with modern showpieces of redwood and glass, all of them darkened by the long shadows of redwoods.

Gabe eased around a hairpin turn and found the mailbox with the number Kate had given him. He pulled in beside her red Saab and got out. He could smell the eucalyptus. A squirrel chattered at him as he climbed the long flight of wooden steps. A hummingbird flitted by, disappearing around the corner of the house.

He rang the bell and waited at the solid mahogany door. He had several minutes to study the landscaping before he heard Kate's voice over the intercom.

"Yes? Who is it?"

"Me. Gabe."

"Hold on. I'll be right out." She appeared at the door a moment later wearing a blue work shirt, white painter's overalls, and soft doeskin moccasins.

"Hi, babes," she said, bending forward to kiss him on the cheek. "Come on in. It's freezing. Is that a suitcase?" She kept her arms folded against the cool evening air. A cat streaked past them, disappearing into the back of the house.

"A briefcase," he said. "I need to show you something."

"Sure. Come on in. I've got a fire going."

A long hallway led to the rear of the house. A Mozart string quartet was playing over a good sound system. He caught a glimpse of a high-ceilinged living room with a large-screen TV. A new Martin guitar lay on a long modern sofa.

She led him into a bright, spacious kitchen with white rafters and track lighting. A log fire burned in a small stone fireplace. A laptop computer stood on the kitchen table, a spreadsheet on the screen, a computer mouse on a red mat beside it. The cat came out from behind the counter and rubbed against Gabe's ankles.

"Great place," he said.

"Yes," Kate said, smiling up at him. "I'm house-sitting for some friends. Ann and Jeremy are in Geneva for a year, doing something for the European Common Market.''

"Lucky you."

She nodded, raising her eyebrows. "Wait till you see the hot tub." A hot bath together had been a regular part of their New Haven routine.

She gestured down at the cat. "This is Sammy. Let me give him his dinner."

She disappeared into the back of the house. Gabe took a seat at the table. A thick book lay beside the computer, *Planning and Financing for the Entrepreneurial Company,* published by Price Waterhouse. A green accountant's pad with long rows of penciled figures lay beside it.

Kate washed out the cat-food can, opened the cabinet under the sink, and dropped it into a tall tub labeled ALUMINIUM ONLY.

Gabe tapped the book with a finger. "Light reading?"

Her face took on a guarded expression. "Just a little project I've been working on. I was going to heat up some pizza. You want some?"

"Sure. I'm starved."

"Help yourself to a beer. You can get me one too."

The refrigerator was full of take-out food in white polyethylene containers. He selected two bottles of Grolsch, opened the fancy ceramic flip-tops, and brought them back to the table, pushing the papers carefully aside.

"Looks like you're up to something, Katie."

"I . . . I don't know," she said. "This is all very confidential."

"If it was really confidential you wouldn't have left it spread out all over the place when you knew I was coming," he said.

"This is true," she said, punching buttons on the microwave. "All right. Hell, why not? I'm trying to buy this bankrupt hot springs up in Sonoma County. I want to turn it into a fitness retreat and workshop center. Here, let me show you."

She sat down in front of the computer, moving and clicking the mouse. The spreadsheet was replaced by rows of tiny icons and file folders. Kate clicked the mouse again.

A digitized black-and-white image of a landscape appeared on the computer screen. Gabe could make out a grove of trees, a range of rolling hills, and a few small buildings.

"There it is," she said, sitting back proudly. "What do you think?"

"You say it has a hot spring?"

"Yep. A hundred and eight degrees, all year round."

Gabe nodded, sipping his beer. He was confused for a moment. Then the light dawned. "A fat farm," he said.

Kate made a face. "Not *just* a fat farm, sweetie. The fat farm to end all fat farms. A place people could come to relax, lose weight, get in shape, have a romantic vacation, or attend a workshop. A romantic inn and health spa with a superb health-food restaurant next door."

"So you're not planning to stay at Kimberley forever."

"Hell no. Another eighteen months, two years, max. But till then I figure I can use all the exposure I can get."

The microwave buzzer went off. She brought the steaming pizza to the table, setting it down with a flourish. It was piled high with vegetables.

"You see before you the full range of my cooking abilities," she said, passing him a plate.

"The permanent clean-up crew, right?" Gabe helped himself to a slice.

She nodded, laughing. "God, yes. I'd forgotten that." Their joint efforts at cooking had been so unsuccessful that their New Haven housemates had prevailed on them to limit themselves to cleaning up.

"So what was it you wanted to show me?"

He looked down at his briefcase. "I really hate to bring it up," he said. It felt wonderful to be there in the kitchen with Kate, eating pizza, hearing about her dream.

"Don't then." Kate lifted a thin piece of pizza to her lips. "We can talk about it later, after we get out of the hot tub."

"I'm afraid I have to. Give me ten minutes, okay?"

She shrugged. "Sure. I can stand anything for ten minutes."

He took out three manila folders. "These are case summaries of three people who died of unexplained hypertensive crisis within the last week. Lindsey and two others—"

"There've been others? How awful."

He reached across the table and put his hand on hers. "Kate. They were all taking Virazine."

"Lindsey was taking Virazine?" she said. Gabe saw the shock and confusion in her eyes.

"Yes. Some idiot of a doctor at San Francisco State gave it to her for a case of mono. On a sales rep's recommendation."

"And you think . . . Oh, come on, Gabe. That's just not possible. This drug has been so well tested—"

He held his hands up in front of him, palms out.

"Hold on," he said. "I'm not saying the drug is responsible."

Her eyes narrowed. "Well what *are* you saying, then?" She pressed her lips together and reached for the folders.

"I'm just saying it needs to be looked into."

"Well, yes. Obviously."

"I was hoping you'd help."

"Of course I'll help." She folded her hands on the table. "What do you want me to do?"

"Take me up to Kimberley tomorrow so I can give them copies and check this thing out."

"Sure. That's no problem." She flipped through one of the folders, an irritated expression on her face. "Tell me about these people," she said.

Gabe brought her up to date on Lindsey's case and took her through what he knew about Juan Rodriguez and Robert Blumberg. She finished her pizza and pushed her plate away.

"Three cases," she said, tapping a pencil against her lip. "Out of what, hundreds of thousands of people who've taken the drug?"

"There may be more," Gabe said. "Do you know if they've received any other adverse-drug-reaction reports?"

She shook her head. "Not that I've heard of. You'd have to ask Arthur McCauley."

"I guess he's the one who should get these copies," Gabe said.

"Yes, unfortunately."

"Why unfortunately?"

Kate rolled her eyes at the ceiling. "You'll see," she said. "He's a stuffy, obnoxious little bear of a man. He has no real power at the company. He's only there because he was a friend of Ed's father. But, Gabe?"

"Yeah?"

"Promise me something: No accusations. No scare headlines. No talking about this to anyone else. Including Ed."

"Kate, give me a break. I'm *trying* to give you guys a chance to prove the drug's okay."

She stuck out her jaw. "I know how involved you get in these things. I want you to promise."

"All right, all right. I promise."

"Thank you. I'll take you up there tomorrow morning. On one condition."

"What now?"

Her eyes met his. The softness had returned to her face. "That we don't have to talk about this any more tonight," she said.

The hot tub was on the hill behind the house. He followed her up the redwood steps, each of them carrying a large colored beach towel. The backyard was screened from the houses on either side by a stepped redwood fence that followed the line of the hillside.

The sun had gone down and it was nearly dark. Small recessed fixtures set into the base of the fence cast soft pools of light. A gentle wind was moving the leaves of the eucalyptus trees.

The tub was set into a redwood deck with a view over the roof of the house to the lights of the valley below. Kate hung her towel on a wooden peg, removed the light foam lid, folded it, and leaned it against the fence. White steam rose from the black water.

"I'm getting in. I'm freezing," she said. She slipped out of her robe, hanging it next to the towel. He caught a fleeting glimpse of her pale torso, her long brown arms and legs. She stepped down onto the bench beneath the water, pausing, thigh-deep, to look back at him over her shoulder.

"It's perfect." She lowered herself slowly until only her head remained above the water's steaming surface. She took a deep breath, held her nose, and disappeared under the water. The deck was suddenly heavy with silence.

Gabe hung up his towel, slipped out of his robe, stepped down onto the underwater wooden bench, then lowered himself slowly until his chin touched the water. Some part of Kate's body brushed lightly against his leg.

The water seemed much too hot. He took several long, slow breaths, relaxing into it, looking out at the lights below.

Kate resurfaced with a splash, her hair plastered back on her head. She smiled across at him, her pale body shimmering under the water.

"Oh, God. It feels so good," she said. "This is my salvation. I come up here just about every night." She moved around the circular bench until she was sitting close beside him. He could feel her body against his, firm and soft and warm. They looked out at the view together.

He nodded. "I can see why. It's so peaceful."

"That's why I want to start the spa," she said. "People *need* a place like this. A little island of peace in a busy life. A place where they can just let everything go, let everything settle down. Tell the whole world to go to hell for a while."

She moved across him to check the thermometer. "A hundred and eight degrees. Just right." She smiled. "So. You ready for the unveiling?"

She rose slowly out of the water. On first glance her breasts looked quite normal. He was mildly surprised.

"They look pretty good to me," he said.

"Look closer."

Her left breast bore several faint scars. There were some changes in coloration due to the skin grafting. There was a strange beauty to it, like some odd tribal markings. The breast itself seemed almost too perfect.

"So that's it, huh?"

"That's it."

"They did a nice job. Barely noticeable, if you ask me."

She nodded. "They used a flap from my abdomen. It's wild. They do it all under a microscope. I got a tummy tuck in the bargain. When I woke up, there it was."

He crossed the tub, raising one hand to each side of her chest.

"You didn't need a tummy tuck," he said.

"Show me the woman who doesn't think she needs a tummy tuck."

Gabe shifted his position. Kate drew in a quick breath as he touched her gently under the water.

"The new one feels a little firmer," he said.

"Scar tissue," she said.

"How does it feel?"

"Some places are still a little numb."

She brought her face close to his. Her breath was coming more quickly now. She lowered herself in the water, bringing her lips down to brush his. He felt the gentle touch of her hand on his hip.

She stood up, laughing, pushing him back to his seat. He could feel her hands on his chest, on his thighs. He bit his bottom lip, leaning his head back against the clean wood of the tank. Kate disappeared under the water. Then he could feel her mouth, gentle, tentative, and tender.

122

She came up smiling, spouting water into the air.

"I've always wanted to do that," she said.

He moved toward her. They kissed, up to their chins in the hot water.

"Here," she said. "Let me float you."

Kate ducked under the water, lifting him easily in her arms. He was floating on his back, looking up at the sky, her right arm under his shoulders, her left supporting his thighs.

"Relax," she said. "I won't let you drown. Relax as much as you can," she said in her workshop-leader's tone. "And pay attention to whatever it is that keeps you from relaxing more."

He lay back in the water, taking long, slow breaths. It felt odd to have her hold him. He felt warm and safe, both vulnerable and protected. It was a pleasant, unfamiliar feeling.

"What's the name of this technique?" he said.

She laughed. "It's called the wellness seduction method."

He nodded lazily, looking up at the sky. "It's very effective," he said.

He woke up later that evening in Kate's heavy brass bed. The rectangular eye of a big-screen Sony TV stared back at him. It was dark outside the window. There was a faint smell of powder in the room. The house was quiet. He sensed that he was alone.

Leaning over her dresser, peering down at the cluttered jars and tubes of makeup, Gabe was stricken by waves of long-forgotten memory: the heavy pots of face cream and the small, shiny bottles of perfume reminded him of his mother's dressing table.

On top of his neatly folded clothes, Gabe found a note: "Had to stop by the office to check a computer run. Help yourself to anything you like. Hit *play* on the VCR in the living room to complete a vital part of your education.'' At the bottom of the note were three small, precisely drawn hearts. He showered, opened a beer, stretched out on the couch, and started the video.

It was a tape of the Atlanta Women's Marathon Classic. The camera operator was in a van that kept just ahead of the leader, a tall, hatchet-faced blond woman with a long, single braid. A second cameraman was in a motorcycle sidecar a few yards ahead of Kate, who trailed the leader by nearly two hundred yards.

Kate was just passing the twenty-five mile mark. She looked back over her shoulder and signaled a stocky young woman who was trailing her on a ten-speed bike. The bicyclist drew up beside Kate and tossed her a water bottle. The announcer predicted that they were about to see the start of the famous Kate Reiley finishing kick.

Kate took a long drink, tossed back the bottle, and gradually began to increase her speed. Gabe could see her stride growing longer. Her arms began to swing back and forth with greater force, her hands grasping the air as if to pull her forward.

The blond woman glanced back over her shoulder. She too lengthened her stride. Kate was gaining, but it would clearly not be enough. She was still fifty yards behind by the time they entered the stadium.

'' . . . And so the great German runner proves again, here in Atlanta, that she is still the the master of the women's marathon, although American new-comer Kate Reiley pressed her all the way, and certainly gave her quite a scare at the end.''

There was a congratulatory interview with the winner. Then the camera cut away to Kate, who was leaning over, her hands on her knees. A blond woman sportscaster, a vaguely familiar veteran of some past Olympics, stepped up and put her blue-blazered arm across Kate's sweat-drenched shoulders, turning her gently to face the camera.

"Kate, you almost got her with that last amazing mile of yours," she said. "Did you wait too long this time? If you had it to do over, would you start your kick back at the twenty-four-mile mark?"

Kate smiled and shook her head. As the camera zoomed in, Gabe saw that she was soaked with perspiration.

"I probably should have tried to keep a little closer when she pulled away from the pack at the fifteen-mile mark, but it was all I could do stay up as close as I did. I was having a little trouble with the heat. But the bottom line was that Maritova ran a great marathon today. I gave it everything I had, but it wasn't quite enough. She deserved to win. I don't think anyone in the world could have caught her today."

"Thanks, Kate. You'll have another shot at Maritova two months from today, in the San Francisco Women's Marathon. The weather should be a little cooler. And NBC will be there. Now back to you, Irv."

Gabe was watching the remaining finishers when the real Kate came in.

"You were looking pretty good there," he said. He reached up and drew her down into his lap.

"Not quite good enough," she said. "Maritova's better than good. Sometimes I think I'll never beat her. Even though I *have* run faster marathons than she has."

"You'll get her next time."

"I hope so. I know I'll probably never be in a category with the really great women's marathoners—Joan Benoit, Grete Waitz, and Ingrid Kristiansen. But I damn well should be able to beat Maritova. My best is nearly two minutes less than the best time she's ever run.''

She shook her head, laughing. "It's odd, isn't it? I *would* pick out a tape where Maritova beats me. You'd think I could at least have left you a video of a race I *won*.''

18

Kimberley Laboratories' headquarters was in northern Marin County, a few miles north of San Rafael. Kate waved to the uniformed guard at the gate and turned up a wide, curving drive. Beds of bright flowers blanketed both sides of the road. There were many acres of well-tended lawn.

They drove through a golf course, passed a cluster of tennis courts, crossed a soft-surfaced running trail, and stopped in front of a massive white stone building, the company headquarters.

"There it is," Kate said. "The space station in the sky." A thick hedge screened the parking garage beneath so that the building seemed to hover high above the ground.

"It's big," Gabe said.

Kate nodded. "Bigger than it looks. Nearly half

the usable space is underground. They say it was under construction for nearly four years."

Kate pulled into a space with her name on it, just inside the garage. She dug a laminated photo ID out of her purse and clipped it to her lapel as they walked to the main entrance. A pale-faced guard affixed a visitor's pass to Gabe's jacket.

They got into the elevator and Kate pushed the button for B-4, the lowest level. She waited until the door closed, then put a hand on Gabe's arm. "I got us here early so I could take you to meet someone. This is all off the record, okay?"

"Sure."

"These people are such tight-asses." She leaned back against the polished oak paneling, holding her black leather briefcase in both hands, swinging it forward and backward. "I could get in a lot of trouble. Especially with this whole Virazine business. But Howard's a great fan of yours. I know he'd love to meet you."

"He's the research guy Dean brought over from Crystal Labs?"

She nodded. "He's a very special person," she said, looking down at the floor. "He helps me keep things in perspective."

They got out on the lower floor. The lights were much dimmer there, the floors a plain gray tile. A series of colored pipes ran along the ceiling. They passed a metal fire door marked ELEVATOR MAINTENANCE, another labeled AIR CONDITIONING. There was a peculiar smell to the place, something between a hospital and an electric generator.

Kate led him to the wide metal door at the end of the hallway. Gabe heard a deep rumbling inside.

"It's a laminar-flow room," Kate said. "We'll need to put on masks and gloves. You remember the standard operating procedure, don't you?" A laminar-flow room is used for people with severe diseases of the immune system. A continuous flow of filtered air passes from one end of the room to the other.

Gabe nodded, putting on a pair of gloves from the shelf beside the door. "Sure. You stay downwind of the patient. So why does Howard need a laminar-flow room?"

"He has AIDS," she said. "And a pretty bad case of juvenile diabetes as well. He's already had one leg amputated—diabetic gangrene—and he's lost most of the feeling in his other leg. He's taking an experimental new Japanese anti-AIDS drug, DPU, once a week. It's working pretty well, but it depresses his immune system for a couple of days each time he takes it. As long as his T-cell count is down, he's very susceptible to infection, so he stays down here in the protected environment. When it's up, we sometimes let him go home."

"The company put in a whole laminar-flow room? Just for this one guy?"

"That's right."

Gabe let out a soft whistle. "Must have cost a bundle."

Kate smiled. "Let me put it this way: We have twenty-two medicinal chemists working full time to come up with new drugs. Right now we have maybe twenty-five new drugs in the research pipeline. Nearly half of them came from Howard."

"I see what you mean. How did he get AIDS?"

"I think he's probably gay," Kate said. "I don't really know for sure. I've never asked. All set?"

"All set."

He followed her into the room. The sound grew louder. A barrier of wide, transparent plastic strips blew up at them, dropping again after Gabe closed the door behind them. He felt a soft, warm draft on his face. Through the trembling plastic strips he saw what appeared to be a large, cluttered office.

"I don't see him," Kate said, lowering her voice. "He must be in the back." She stepped through the plastic curtain, motioning Gabe to remain where he was.

He stood with his hands behind him, looking in through the swaying plastic curtain. He could make out a computer workstation with a large color screen. A floor-to-ceiling bookshelf held an untidy assortment of books, reference manuals, and stacks of journals. A miniature basketball hoop hung at eye level. Beside it was a large poster with a black-and-white picture of Albert Einstein sticking out his tongue. Some of the desks were fitted with large metal shutters, like oversized music stands. Gabe decided that they must be windscreens.

He heard Kate calling over the noise of the fans. A few minutes later a smiling youth with a mustache rolled his wheelchair into the room. He was much younger than Gabe had expected. Kate leaned forward to speak to him, as a fond mother might lean down to talk to a child. She gestured back in Gabe's direction. Howard held up a hand in greeting, his handsome face transfigured with delight. He said something to Kate, listened to her response, then threw his head back and laughed up at the ceiling. The sound of his laugher rose above the steady hum of the fans.

Kate looked back at Gabe, beckoning him to join them. The wind was stronger inside the plastic curtain. Howard wheeled up to Gabe, his hand extended, grinning merrily. His right leg was missing, his forehead lightly beaded with perspiration, his cheeks slightly sunken. But his face was charged with good humor and enthusiasm. He was wearing a Grateful Dead T-shirt.

"Howard. Careful!" Kate barked a sharp warning. She backed toward the door so as to stay downwind of him.

"Sorry. I keep forgetting." Howard dropped his hand to his lap, screwing up his face in a comic expression of mock frustration. His long, handsome face was flushed with excitement. He could have been a graduate student or an intense young rabbi.

"Gabe Austin, Howard Pearlman," Kate said.

"It's great to meet you, sir," he said. Howard's face seemed to shine with a biblical glow. "I got all excited when Kate said you were a friend of hers. I've been watching you on TV for a long time."

"Howard is one of our top researchers," Kate said, positioning herself protectively beside him. "And a very good friend."

"I taped your series on AIDS," Howard said. "I've been showing it to some friends of mine. It's really quite lovely."

"Howard is working on some ideas for a new drug treatment for AIDS," Kate said.

"Really?" Gabe asked. "What are you doing?"

"Just the same old thing," Howard said. "Tweaking and twining." He smiled shyly, looking down at his hands. "I feel so lucky they were willing to build this room for me. And now I have Dr. Reiley taking such good care of me."

"A cure for AIDS," Gabe said. "That would be quite an accomplishment."

Howard shrugged. "It'd be too late for me, of course. But it'd be a nice little thank-you note to leave behind. I've had a great response to DPU. If I'm lucky I might have another good year or even two." He smiled. "You can do a hell of a lot in a year. Did you know Mozart wrote twenty-two major pieces the year he was my age?'' Gabe swallowed hard. There was something about Howard that made him think of some inspired Old Testament prophet.

"How did you come up with riboxyuridine?" Gabe asked.

"Virazine? Oh, that was easy," Howard said. "I started with the acyclovir molecule and just tweaked a few pieces around."

"Tweaked?"

Howard nodded toward the computer. "Yep. On this little baby right here."

"I'd like to see how you did that."

"Here, let me show you." Howard rolled his chair toward the machine. The screen displayed a color image of a complex organic molecule.

"This is the drug I'm playing with right now," Howard said. "Let's say we want to pop off a hydrogen and put on an acetyl group." He bent over the keyboard, his fingers flying, then sat back and gave the return key a satisfied whack. One of the small blue spheres faded away. A larger cluster, a lumpy pyramid in light green, appeared in its place. The big molecule shifted its shape slightly to accommodate it. Howard pressed another series of keystrokes and the molecule began turning slowly before their eyes.

"There are basically two ways you can design a new drug on a computer," he said.

"Even I know that." Kate smiled. "You can tweak or you can twine."

"Right," Howard said. "You can start with an active molecule and tweak it around until you get something interesting. Or you can start with the receptor site and build a molecule that will twine itself right into it. We actually ran into some pretty interesting things about Virazine in the computer model . . ."

Kate cleared her throat, taking a step forward. "That's going to have to wait," she said. "We're due upstairs. Howard? Have you had your insulin shot?"

Howard shook his head. An uneasy expression passed across his face. "I . . . No. I've been kind of busy."

She nodded understandingly. "Want me to do it?"

Howard suddenly looked sulky, irresolute. "Yeah, I guess." He looked hopelessly up at Gabe. "It's such a hassle," he said. "And since I'm sick I have to scrub before I do it. It's such a drag. It's nice to have someone else do it for me once in a while."

"Where do you want it?" Kate was gentle but resolute.

"My left arm, I guess."

They moved to the low counter against the wall. Kate cleaned the injection site with alcohol swabs. She then took off her gloves, scrubbed her hands at a low sink, and put on a new pair of gloves. Gabe smiled to himself. Most physicians he knew put on two or three pairs of gloves when giving an AIDS patient an injection. Following her instructions, he swabbed the top of the insulin vial and held it upside down while she drew the clear liquid up into the syringe.

"So. What do you think?" Kate said as they waited for the elevator.

Gabe shook his head. "Tweaking and twining. Jesus." The elevator doors opened and he followed her in.

"He's quite a guy," Kate said. She took Gabe's arm, leaning against him as the elevator started up. "You've got to keep this visit completely confidential. Okay?"

"Sure," Gabe said.

"I could get into a lot of trouble. That's all top-secret stuff he's working on." She glanced at her watch. "I'm running late. If you don't mind, we'll cut through the production area."

They left the elevator on the next floor up. Kate inserted her card in the slot next to a pair of automatic doors that read PRODUCTION AREA—EMPLOYEES ONLY. The doors opened and they stepped through into one end of a long, air-conditioned hallway with high ceilings and sparkling white walls.

"This is a clean area," Kate said. "We need to put on masks and gowns and shoe covers."

"You're sure this is all right?" Gabe said.

"Oh, sure. Everyone uses it all the time. The hallway is no big deal. The real clean areas are behind those windows."

They helped themselves to gowns and gloves and masks. Small groups of workers, similarly garbed, passed them in the hallway, using their identity cards to open the sliding electric doors that led to the various production areas.

Gabe and Kate made their way down the central hallway, looking in at the quiet assembly lines, the still, silent rows of pill-making machines.

"So this is where they make all those pills," Gabe said.

"This is where," Kate said. "This line on the left is for Ulcid, our antiulcer drug. The one on the right makes our new line of dog and cat flea collars."

"Flea collars," Gabe said. "Isn't that an unusual product for a drug company?"

"It's highly unusual," Kate said. "Most pharmaceutical companies make only prescription drugs. But Ed has decided to go after the direct-to-the-consumer market as well. We've built a whole separate sales force to handle our over-the-counter products."

Gabe looked in at the moving belt behind the window. "It looks like it's already running," he said.

Kate nodded. "It's almost completely automated. Howard and Gertrude came up with a new high-pressure process to put the active ingredient into a special slow-release plastic-resin matrix. It's given us a big advantage over our competition."

"That's right. I remember her telling me about it." Gabe was studying a warning sign taped to the window. "I can't believe you've got nerve gas floating around in there," he said.

"Actually, at very small doses, it's practically harmless to humans," she said. "The levels inside are low enough to be completely filtered out by the suits our inspectors wear. See?" She pointed at two figures in shiny spaceman outfits. They were wearing shiny helmets and bulky backpacks.

"Those are our quality control inspectors," Kate said. "The production line is completely automated so they only have to go in twice a day. But there's a bit of the active ingredient released when the collars are cut, and there's always the risk of a leak from the kettles." She pointed up at three massive stainless steel vats. "Without the filtration units, that could be a real disaster."

They discarded their masks and gowns at the far end of the hallway. A long, bright passage led them into another section of the headquarters complex. Kate took him down a carpeted hallway, through a door marked FITNESS CENTER, and into a quiet reception area with comfortable chairs and couches, magazines, telephones, and soft classical music. A hallway to one side led to the men's and women's locker rooms. Through the wide double doors straight ahead Gabe saw a huge, high-ceilinged room full of exercise equipment.

A trim gray-haired woman in a black running suit was tapping away at a computer terminal behind the counter.

"So, Lucy, anything pressing?"

"Hi, Dr. Reiley. Not really. Your mail and your calls are in on your desk. You're taking Bridgette's noon aerobics class today. And the big boss wants you to bring Dr. Austin by to say hello. He's down on court one."

Kate's inner office was a cheery windowless room with white walls, light gray carpets, and large abstract posters of sporting scenes. An exercise bike stood next to a motorized treadmill.

"Your own private gym," Gabe said.

"Practically." She stepped behind her desk, leaning down to scan her messages. Gabe stepped up on the treadmill. A copy of *Runner's World* was clipped to the reading rack. A telephone headset lay on a high table.

"Give me just a minute to confirm your meeting with Arthur," she said.

"No problem." He braced himself on the metal rail and pushed the button that turned on the motor. The wide black belt began to move slowly beneath his feet. He pulled back on the stainless steel speed-control lever. He had to walk faster to keep from being swept off the machine.

Kate put down the receiver. "All set," she said. "Come on, I'll give you the grand tour."

Two dozen Nautilus machines were arranged in a large rectangle in the middle of the room. Two men and a woman, all wearing blue shorts and white T-shirts with blue Kimberley logos, made their way from one machine to the next, adjusting the weight stacks, climbing on, doing their ten or twelve repetitions, making a check on a small blue clipboard. A wide jogging lane ran around the outside of the room. A thick-set woman with shiny hand weights and a choppy, determined stride had it all to herself.

"Quite a setup," Gabe said.

Kate nodded. "Ed has been very supportive," she said. "And we've been getting great results."

A row of six exercise bikes stood in the center of the room, each equipped with a small TV with earphones and a reading rack. A friendly woman with warm brown eyes and graying hair waved to Kate. She was watching a gardening video. A tall, thin woman with a sweat band was reading *The Wall Street Journal*. A balding man with earphones pedaled with eyes closed, listening to some inaudible music. The only sound was the whir of flywheels and the occasional clash of weight stacks across the room.

Kate led him along the glass back wall. There were two tennis courts on the floor below. A man in a white tennis hat was practicing his serve. The glass wall on the left looked out over an Olympic-size pool where two women in goggles were swimming laps. A bit farther along they stopped to watch six men playing a half-court game on a full-size basketball court.

She led Gabe through a red metal door and along a dim walkway with a high white railing on each side. The place was full of a popping sound like the echo of small arms fire. Gabe looked down over the railing. Two young women were playing a hard-fought point in the racquetball court below. Kate was at the far end of the walkway, calling down to someone in one of the courts. She beckoned to Gabe to join her.

Ed Elias and Dean Storch looked up from the bright white squash court. Both were wearing Kimberley T-shirts. Elias looked fresh, solid, and trim. Storch had sweated through his shirt and was breathing hard. He leaned against the wall, waved his racquet, and gave them his crooked smile.

"Hello there, Doctor," Elias boomed, his voice echoing in the small, bare space. "I'm glad we were finally able to get you down here. Looks like I might get a decent game of squash today after all."

Kate took Gabe down to the men's locker room and waited outside while he changed. Ten minutes later, wearing a mismatched outfit he had scrounged from the lost and found, Gabe knocked on the squash-court door. *Like a lamb to the slaughter,* he thought. But Elias had promised that in exchange for a few quick games of squash, he would give him an on-the-record interview.

Elias opened the door, shook Gabe's hand, made a comical comment on his outfit, and excused himself, leading Kate to a hurried stand-up conference down the hall. Gabe found Storch inside, leaning against the wall. He held out a sweaty hand.

"Getting too damn old for this sort of thing," he said, gasping. His legs were shaking. He looked exposed and vulnerable, like some pale creature pulled unwillingly from its shell. A small paunch bulged over his trunks. Gabe had a sudden impulse to wrap him up in a blanket.

"Deano," Gabe said. "You look kind of beat. You feeling all right?"

"Oh, hell yes. I'm just out of my league." He put out a hand to lean against the wall.

Gabe lowered his voice. "Look. I need to talk to you," he said. "It looks like there may be a major problem with Virazine."

"Oh?" Storch's eyebrows shot up. He frowned in sudden concern. "What kind of a problem?"

Gabe heard Elias's voice outside the door. "I'll talk to you later," he said.

"Yes, certainly," Storch said. "Come up to my office when you're finished with Ed," Storch said. "We'll have lunch. I'll fix it up." Elias was coming back onto the court. Storch reached out to shake Gabe's hand.

"And watch out for his backhand lobs," Storch said.

It proved to be good advice. Gabe was twenty years younger and a good bit quicker, but it didn't seem to matter. Elias kept him running. He could hit a perfect kill shot from nearly anywhere on the court. There was no chitchat. Just Ed's voice calling out the score, the sound of the hard little ball echoing off the walls, and the soft thud as it fell dead and unplayable a few inches from the front wall. In their three games, Gabe scored 6, 4, and 7 points to Ed's winning 21.

19

A glass display case was set into the wall of the waiting area in Ed Elias's office. It held a display of Kimberley milestones: generic aspirin and penicillin; Estriol, an early birth control pill; Kentek, a high blood pressure medication; Ulcid, an antiulcer drug; Wormex, a home veterinary product; the company's dog and cat flea collars; and Virazine, the company's first antiviral. Gabe, fresh from his shower in the locker room downstairs, peered in at the samples dramatically presented on black velvet.

"Dr. Austin?"

"Yes?" Gabe turned to find a petite, energetic young woman in a tweed jacket and bolo tie. She had permed chestnut hair and an offhand air of girlish competence.

"I'm Rebecca, Mr. Elias's personal assistant." Her hand was firm and friendly. "Mr. Elias is running a little behind. He thought you might want to take a quick look at our new video on the history of the company."

Gabe glanced back at the display case. "I'll bet he's in working on the next Kimberley milestone," he said.

Her laugh made the receptionist look up from her computer. "I certainly hope so," Rebecca said. "We could use it."

Gabe followed her down a long, carpeted hallway, past colorful outer offices where secretaries in bright silk blouses guarded the executives within. It was quieter here. The desks were larger, the ceilings higher, the offices more spacious. Gabe was aware that he was among the select.

Rebecca left him in a well-appointed conference room with a remote control and a fresh cup of coffee in an English china cup and saucer. The video on the monitor presented Kimberley Laboratories as a great American success story: Joseph Elias, a penniless immigrant, had come to the United States during the Depression. He had worked for the Bayer company in Italy before the war and had dreams of starting a drug company in his adopted country. He started out making generic aspirin in his basement. From these humble beginnings, through hard work and a keen intellect . . . and so on.

In 1960, Kimberley Laboratories became the first drug company to bring a birth control pill to the U.S. market. The original stockholders had seen their investments increase more than a hundredfold. Gabe was ten minutes into the tape when he was interrupted by a soft knock.

"Hello there, old man. I see Lord Edward is keeping you in his on-deck circle." Storch lowered himself into the adjacent chair, clicked the monitor to mute, and let out a long sigh. The video played on silently on the big screen.

"That's Sheila's little brainchild," he said. "Horatio Alger. The holy family. The whole bit. So what's this about a problem with Virazine?"

"I've got three deaths from uncontrollable hypertensive crisis in people taking your drug."

"Really." Storch looked alarmed. "Does Arthur McCauley know about this?"

"Not yet. I have an appointment to see him at one-thirty."

Storch nodded, his lips pressed tightly together. "And how did you—" He broke off suddenly. Gabe turned to see Rebecca at the door.

"Oh, hello, Dr. Storch," she said. "Excuse me. Dr. Austin, Mr. Elias will see you whenever you're ready."

Storch stood up. "I won't keep you," he said. "Come by when you get through. I'm right down the hall. We'll see what Antoine has cooked up for us over in the executive dining room."

The walls of Elias's office were paneled in hand-rubbed blond oak. There were leather-bound books and paintings of racehorses and fox hunts. A log fire burned in a small stone fireplace.

A large, somber oil painting showed what appeared to be a taller, older version of Elias in an old-fashioned suit, a black Labrador sleeping at his feet. Joseph Elias appeared to be looking down disapprovingly at his grandson. Elias, coatless, was working at a large library table across from the blazing fireplace.

"Come in, come in," Elias said. "Here, give me your jacket. Those were some great games." He took Gabe's coat and waved him to a seat on a pair of couches that faced each other across a heavy glass-topped table.

"I wasn't much competition, I'm afraid."

"You're plenty of competition for me." A wry look passed across Elias's face. Gabe had the unmistakable impression that he was making a veiled reference to Kate. They looked at each other in silence.

A gaunt young man in a double-breasted suit brought in a tray with two glasses, an ice bucket, and a bottle of Italian mineral water. Elias sat on the opposite couch and used silver tongs to drop ice cubes into two glasses.

"Well. I promised you an interview," he said, suddenly all business again. "Here's what I propose: Three questions of your choice. No restrictions. I get as much time as I want to answer. Then we go off the record and talk about the interesting stuff. Fair enough?" He handed Gabe the glass.

"Fair enough." Gabe opened his briefcase, took out his pocket tape recorder, flipped it on, and placed it on the table. "All set?"

Elias smiled. "Fire away."

"Okay. Question number one," Gabe said. "You've had a major, across-the-board price increase on most of your products within the last year. Some of your drugs now cost the patient hundreds of dollars a month. Yet, many of them cost just pennies a pill to make. Are you simply charging as much as the traffic will bear, or is there another, more charitable explanation?''

Irritation flickered in Elias's eyes, but he recovered quickly. "Christ, you go right for the jugular, don't you?''

"You limit me to three questions, I'm going to use them.''

Elias gave him a bemused look. "The cost of research is absolutely killing us. It can easily cost us millions of dollars just to bring a new drug to animal testing. If the rats die, that money goes down the toilet. That means that the drugs that *do* get approved have to help take up the slack. So it's not really fair to look at our unit costs while ignoring our research expenses.

"And as the FDA takes longer and longer to approve a drug for sale, they leave us less and less time to recover our investment. Once the patent expires, the generic-drug companies can legally rip off all our expensive research. It's the biggest problem we face.''

"Okay. Question number two," Gabe said. "What's the *next* biggest problem facing your company today?''

Elias looked down as if he hoped to read the answer in the carpet beneath the table. "Well, I suppose I would again have to go back to the question of research productivity. We're investing heavily in computer-aided drug modeling. And we're looking at ways of giving our research people some kind of ownership in the new drugs they develop. It seems to be working. We have some very exciting new drugs in the pipeline.''

"Last question," Gabe said. "What's the *best* thing that's happened for your company this year?"

Elias smiled. "Our new flea collar is selling nearly four times our most optimistic projections. And we've just introduced our first antiviral drug."

Gabe nodded, biting his lip. He wondered how Elias would respond to the copies of the three medical records in his briefcase.

"And we discovered that our antihypertensive drug Kentek also helps reduce prostate enlargement," Elias continued. "That was a real break. We're filing a new drug application. But since it's already been approved for another use, we won't have to go back and prove it's safe again. That'll save us sixty to eighty million dollars right there. And as the drug is already on the market, we're beginning to see a nice sales increase due to off-label prescribing in advance of FDA approval."

Elias dug into his pocket and wiped his lips with a white handkerchief. "That's your three questions. How'd I do?"

"Not bad. Not bad at all." Gabe turned off his tape recorder and dropped it into his pocket. "I'll give you a chance to read my column before it runs."

"Thank you." Elias smiled, glancing down at his watch. "I appreciate that. Now—I have a conference call in twenty minutes. In the time we have left, I'd like to explore the possibility of you and Kimberley joining forces." Elias leaned forward in his chair, lacing his fingers together.

"We've been monitoring your column and your TV spots for more than a year now. You come across as a man of knowledge and integrity. I don't agree with everything you say, but we do approve of the general thrust of your work. You're clearly in the consumer health education business. We're very interested in that business."

"I thought you were in the business of selling drugs."

"No." Elias shook his head. "That's the short-term view. Our long-term goal is to help people deal with their health needs. I'm convinced that over the next two or three decades the consumer will be playing a larger role in diagnosing his own problems and prescribing his own therapies."

Gabe smiled. "That's supposed to be *my* line."

"Exactly." Elias looked up at the painting over the fireplace. "My grandfather was a great believer in wonder drugs. I've come to believe that the most important thing is how we take care of ourselves. I spend a lot of time in the gym, and I've been surprised at how much I've learned about my body. I think that's going to be the new dimension of health care in the future—the informed, concerned patient. That's one reason we're trying to bring your friend Kate into top management."

"So you're interested in going beyond the prescription-drug business."

Elias nodded. "We've had extraordinary results from our new over-the-counter division, especially with Cortiderm and Tolamine. We've seen what can happen when a drug is switched from prescription-only to OTC status. One of our long-term goals is to buy up the rights to other companies' lackluster prescription drugs, then take them over-the-counter. We'd like to become the industry leader in this type of switch-product."

"Smart," Gabe said.

"Thank you. We're also developing a new line of vitamins. They'll use a new laser technology delivery system that will allow people to take just one pill a week and get greater effectiveness with fewer side effects. And we're exploring the possibility of getting into the health information business in a big way. That's where we need your help."

Elias frowned. "We'd like to start by putting out a patient instruction booklet with each drug we produce." He swirled the ice in his glass. "Our studies tell us consumers want a hell of a lot more information than their doctors give them. You're a pioneer in this field. You've been turning out some high-quality drug information with very little funding and support. Have you ever wondered what you could do with a budget of three or four million dollars a year?"

Gabe stopped in mid-swallow. It was only with great difficulty that he managed to keep from sputtering out his mouthful of mineral water. "What kinds of things are you thinking of?"

Elias shrugged. "You tell us. Audiotext. Videotext. CD-ROM. In-store information systems. Books. Magazines. Newsletters. Cable TV. Video disc. Electronic books. Video cassette. TV syndication. Computer networks. We're wide open at this point. I see people like you and Kate as the new experts. We'd like to have you tell us what you think we should do. Would you be willing to think about that?"

"You make it sound pretty tempting," Gabe said. "But I have to be careful that it doesn't constitute a conflict of interest."

Elias put down his drink and leaned forward. "We might start by having you up for a series of consulting visits, meeting with various members of our staff. It'd give us a chance to get to know each other. We normally pay our top consultants five thousand dollars a day."

The intercom buzzed. "Mr. Elias? Your Paris call is on line three."

Elias put his hand on Gabe's shoulder, leading him to the door. "Think about it," he said. "Talk it over with Dean and with Kate. I've asked Rebecca to introduce you to Chip Downey, our chief of corporate security. He should be able to speed things along." He gave Gabe his hand. "I'll look forward to our next meeting," he said. "And thanks for the game. I know I'm not going to get off so easily next time."

He turned back toward the fireplace and picked up the phone. *"Allo, Jacques? Comment ça va? Eh, bien. Alors, qu'est-ce qui se passe?"*

20

Rebecca was waiting for him in Elias's outer office. "I understand you may be working with us," she said. "Mr. Elias has asked me to help take care of some of the administrative details. And Mr. Brody asked me to give you this." She handed Gabe a manila envelope.

He looked down at the return address. "This is from Ray Brody?" Brody was a well-known San Francisco power broker, a notoriously tough lawyer who was famous for defending major Hollywood studios, drug-dealing celebrities, deposed dictators, and palimony girlfriends. Rumor had it that if you needed a favor from anyone of significance in the San Francisco Bay Area, Ray Brody was the person who could get it for you.

Rebecca nodded. "He's a special consultant to our corporate counsel," she said. "If you'll come this way, I'll take you down to Mr. Downey's office." She took Gabe down to the fifth floor, deposited him at Downey's door, and hurried back to the elevator like a first-class passenger who had mistakenly wandered into the economy cabin.

Gabe sat in Downey's outer office, flipping through a copy of *Corporate Security Today*. For a minute, Elias's proposition had sounded immensely attractive. He saw now why Kate had been so eager for them to meet.

Gabe knew that Sid Crowell, the irascible chief of medicine, was looking for a workable pretense to drop him from the ER rotation at the hospital. Their latest run-in regarding Crowell's liver study had made that only too plain. Consulting for Kimberley would help cover him financially if Crowell got his way.

But would they still want him after he showed Arthur McCauley the three case reports? And how would working for Kimberley affect his ability to find a solution to the Virazine problem? He reminded himself that had not agreed to anything yet.

Downey was a large, solid, smiling man with a gray-white flat-top. From the look on his face, he had a lot of things on his mind, none of them good. He was sitting beneath a wall covered with framed diplomas, awards, and certificates. He held a glowing cigarette cupped in his hand as if to keep it as far from his visitor as possible. He seemed preoccupied, troubled, and strangely sympathetic.

"Dr. Austin. A pleasure, sir." He put out the cigarette in a metal wastebasket and came around his desk. He was a full head taller than Gabe. His fingers were as big as sausages. It looked as if his barber did most of his work with an electric clipper.

"You'll have to excuse me," he said, waving a hand to blow the smoke away. "These damn things . . . I don't know what it is. . . . Here, sit down, sit down."

The telephone rang. Downey picked it up, settled himself in his oversized leather chair, and ran his hand absently over the top of his head. Several tubes of lip balm and a pack of Vantage Filters lay among the empty Styrofoam cups on his large mahogany desk. Downey looked naggingly familiar. Gabe was sure that he had seen his picture on some sports page, long ago.

Then Downey laughed and barked into the phone and Gabe remembered: Down-Boy Downey had been an all-pro linebacker for the Chicago Bears. The nickname had come from an act he and his teammates performed for the TV cameras: Downey would play the mad dog, barking and snapping from the sidelines, antagonizing the opposing quarterback during the pregame warm-up. His teammates would hold him back by his jersey, shouting, "Down, boy, down, boy!" Downey had gone to jail for contempt of court after refusing to testify in a point-shaving scam.

Downey finished his phone call and folded his big hands on the desk like a man forcing himself to forgo a pleasant chat in the name of business. "Ed thinks you're going to be just the ticket for the consulting job he's been trying to fill," he said. "He's asked me to get the ball rolling. It's pretty routine. We do it for all our employees and consultants. I believe Rebecca gave you a copy of our confidentiality form?"

"She gave me something—from Ray Brody, no

less." Gabe took the envelope out of his briefcase and dropped it on Downey's desk.

"You know Ray?"

"Only by reputation."

Downey nodded patiently. "I wouldn't worry too much about it. This has to go through our legal department." Downey opened the envelope and took out the computer-printed form. "It's your basic consulting contract with some security provisions thrown in. All standard information—social security, driver's license, military record, employment history. Just a formality, really."

"Nobody's offered me a job yet."

"Well, just between you and me, Ed's talking like it's a sure thing." Downey looked down at the paper like a man looking at his income tax form. "The big boss likes to move fast, and these things can take two or three weeks to clear. Shame to hold up important business, you know what I mean?"

Downey's phone rang again. He picked it up, spoke briefly, and covered the receiver with a thick hand. "I'm afraid I need to take this call," he said, glancing down at the paper on the desk. "You can go ahead and read this over and sign it. Just leave it on the desk outside."

"I'll take it along," Gabe said, picking up the form. He stood up. "If Ed and I come to some agreement, I'll fill it out and bring it by."

Storch's office was back upstairs, just down the hall from Ed's. It looked like a room in the Museum of Modern Art.

Storch was sitting behind a slab of ebony marble supported by gleaming stainless-steel pillars. There were two computers on the credenza behind him. A black marble conference table and a half dozen padded leather chairs stood across the room. In its own way, the office was as large and as spectacular as Ed's.

Storch stubbed out his cigarette in a heavy glass ashtray and raised a welcoming hand. "Johnny, I'm going to put you on hold for just a second." He pushed a button, put down the receiver, and came around his desk. His handshake was solid and he looked quite himself again, safe once more in his London-tailored suit, the haggard but thoughtful—and slightly ironic—elder statesman.

"Come in. Come in. I see you survived your encounter with Lord Edmund."

"Yes. But I'm afraid my pride didn't," Gabe said.

Storch gave him a sad, knowing smile. "You get used to that. Listen, I need another minute or two on the phone. Phyllis will get you coffee if you like." He put a friendly hand on Gabe's shoulder, walking him toward the back of the room. "There are a few paintings in the alcove back there you might enjoy. You don't mind amusing yourself for a few minutes?"

Storch returned to his desk and continued his conversation. "Well, what is this guy's problem anyway?" Storch was saying. The British accent had gone out of his voice. It was quite midwestern now. "My God, man, you've got to *lean* on this guy. Yes, whatever it takes." Gabe glanced back at his friend. He was sitting behind his desk, reaching for a cigarette from the gold box on the credenza. He lit it with a silver desk lighter, blowing a plume of white smoke up over his head.

"We can't put up with any more of this," Storch was saying. "Let's keep it simple. He misses one more deadline, his days of sucking on the corporate tit are over for good."

In the far corner, behind a lacquered Chinese

screen, Gabe found a small private sitting area with a gray leather sofa, an easy chair, and a dozen closely hung paintings. The first was a small Picasso drawing, a nude sitting on a stool with her arms behind her. Next to the Picasso was a small, colorful oil of an open window by Paul Signac. Farther along the wall he discovered two small Matisse seascapes. Gabe looked at them closely. They all appeared to be originals. He raised his eyebrows. Dean had come a long way from his organic-chemistry lab at Berkeley.

Gabe had first visited Storch's Berkeley lab halfway through Gabe's sophomore year. Storch was a brilliant but eccentric young faculty member with shoulder-length hair, an ex–Rhodes Scholar who wore a black leather jacket and drove a supercharged Austin-Healey on the amateur racing circuit. He was feared by his students. It was said that he could be found, day or night, in his laboratory on the top floor of the old chemistry building. And so, one rainy day in January, Gabe had made his way up the three flights of worn stone stairs.

Gabe knocked on the laboratory door, received no answer, walked in, and found himself in a dim, high-ceilinged room filled with battered black lab benches stacked with beakers, bottles, and other pieces of chemical apparatus. Gabe walked through the room to the back and knocked at an inner office door. Again he received no answer. He pushed it open and looked in. A tall, dark figure stood at a large wooden easel, totally absorbed in a wild, bright canvas. The artist, a ghostly long-haired man, wore a tattered white lab coat over a black turtleneck. A Mozart piano concerto was playing on a battered record player.

Gabe stood silently, watching the man paint. There was a fascinating intensity about the way he moved.

The painting, which must have been at least four feet square, was an interlocking assemblage of what appeared to be devils and angels. The devils, red and black, grinned like satyrs. The angels' robes were gold and white, their faces transfixed in the most pious of expressions. It was as though they were doing some wild line dance, angels and devils together.

Gabe stood in the doorway for fifteen minutes before the older man noticed him. He let out a grunt like a displeased bear, threw his brush and palate on a low work table, and charged across the room.

"Out, damn you. Can't you see I'm in the middle of something? Out. Out. I'll be with you in a bit."

Gabe waited in the outer laboratory. Half an hour later Storch came storming out. He washed his hands in a filthy black sink and lit a Pall Mall.

"All right. What is it?" Storch must have been about forty, his long hair streaked with gray. He was tall and thin, rather ascetic-looking, with a prominent pale forehead, gold-rimmed glasses, and stained yellow teeth. Gabe introduced himself and said that he would like to register for Storch's advanced organic-chemistry class.

"Oh you would, would you?" Storch wiped his hands on a dirty towel. He asked some perfunctory questions about the courses Gabe had taken. He seemed amused at Gabe's answers.

"You think you can handle Organic Chemistry 102 without taking 101? Your arrogance is impressive. What makes you think you'll be able to keep up?"

Gabe explained that he had already read the first four chapters of the textbook and had read through a friend's notes for the first semester's lectures. He mentioned that he'd been first in his class in freshman honors chemistry and suggested that Storch might check with his professor.

Storch took an angry puff and shook his head. "I wouldn't trouble myself to speak to that oaf." He searched Gabe's face again with those deep-set, slightly protruding gray eyes. "All right. I'll let you in. You might just brighten up that dim-witted class of mine."

Gabe had done so well that when Storch had gone to Washington to give a paper six weeks later, he'd asked Gabe to take over the class. There was some grumbling among the other pre-med students, but most of them preferred Gabe to Storch.

"Look, old man," Storch said when he came back. "You're so far ahead of those other poor dolts. How'd you like to be my unofficial TA? You really do learn more by teaching, you know, if you can stand it. And maybe you can figure out something you'd like to try to make in the lab."

And so Gabe had gone to work in Storch's laboratory. It was his introduction to pharmacology. Unlike most organic chemists, Storch kept up with the latest developments in pharmacology and molecular biology. He was a hard worker, toiling in his lab from 5:00 A.M. till lunchtime, teaching in the afternoons and putting in long hours in his painting studio each evening. When Gabe discovered that Storch was selling his paintings through a San Francisco gallery under his real name, Dino Storchiani, the older man shrugged it off.

"Peanuts," he said. "The gallery gets most of it. I make ten times as much with these." He showed him a selection of tubes marked with drug company identification codes. Storch was making small batches of experimental drugs for several pharmaceutical companies.

The Dean Storch that Gabe had found at Yale three years later was a different man. He had shaved off his mustache, gotten a haircut, and was buying his clothes at J. Press. He was running his own laboratory—with a complement of graduate students and post-docs. He was genial, funny, and self-deprecating. And he could drink a glass of sherry with the best of them.

It was clear from the beginning that continuing his friendship with Gabe, a lowly medical student, would have been an embarrassment to an up-and-coming junior faculty member. Once Gabe began working in Gertrude's lab he couldn't help running into Storch in the halls. They slapped each other on the back and spoke of getting together. But they never did.

Halfway through Gabe's second year of medical school Storch showed up at the Edgewood house late at night. He was quite drunk. A large grant had come through—half a million dollars to attempt the synthesis of a new neurotransmitter that had been isolated from human brain tissue. The award had led to a fight with the chairman of the pharmacology department, an owlish man named Gatzberg. Dr. Gatzberg, who had opposed the grant proposal, now demanded to be credited as a co-investigator. Unless he did, Gatzberg had made it clear, Storch could kiss any hopes of tenure goodbye.

Gabe's housemates were out. They sat on the battered couch while Storch refilled their glasses from a magnum of Italian Chianti.

"Wastin' my fuckin' life in that bloody laboratory, anyway," he said. "Should have stuck with my painting. Might have been a halfway decent artist by now."

Gabe remembered the vibrant canvases from the

lab at Berkeley. "How did you get started painting?" he asked.

"A wonderful old don at Oxford. Years ago. Art history professor. Made students go out with brushes and paints. Amateur painter himself. Became rather obsessed with it. Took a year out to paint and study in Florence and Paris."

"Why'd you give it up?"

"Got to know some real artists." Storch rolled his eyes at the ceiling. "Bunch of old men sitting around in their pee-stained underwear, complaining how unappreciated they were. Some of them better painters than I'll ever be. Man's got to be tough. Bite the bullet. Do what has to be done. You know what I need to do now?"

Gabe shook his head.

Storch refilled his glass and let out a long belch. "Gotta go 'pologize to Dr. Gasbag. Invite him to be my co-fucking-investigator." Storch finished the wine, took a deep drag on his cigarette, and stubbed it out. "Have to set things up first. Worst thing you can do. 'Pologize when a chap's not expecting it. Mind if I practice a 'pology or two on you?"

Gabe invited him to go ahead.

Storch leaned forward on the couch and waved a finger at Gabe. "Hey, Dr. Gasbag. I apologize, you crap-brained little chicken-fart. I would just love to have your fucking scrawny ass as my co-investigator. You hear me, you dumb fuck? I'm a bull-headed dago. Grave character defects and all that." He showed Gabe his crooked yellow teeth. " 'Pologizing for fun and profit," he said. "I should go on the goddamn circuit."

Two days later Storch went to Dr. Gatzberg's office and apologized. Dr. Gatzberg agreed to become his co-investigator. Storch never *was* able to synthesize the polypeptide, but neither was anyone else. It was someone in Gertrude's lab who had told Gabe that Storch had left Yale to enter Stanford Business School.

Gabe was still looking dreamily up at the paintings when he realized that Storch had finished his conversation and was standing beside him.

"You've gone back to your old love, I see," Gabe said.

Storch shook his head, smiling. "Oh, no. Just a lowly collector." He smiled, leaning forward to look at the paintings. "It's my one indulgence, old man. My one weakness." He reached up to touch a simple wood frame.

"They're really quite something," Gabe said.

"Yes. And do you know that no one around here has ever noticed them? Except for our controller, who can't understand why our insurance premiums are so high. I'm considered a wild eccentric around here. Even then it might not be so bad—if Ed Elias only knew what he was doing." He shook his head sadly. "The man has no sense of what it takes to do drug research. Or how to really push a new drug. But you didn't come to hear my problems. Let's eat."

The executive dining room was on the top floor of the Kimberly building and had a panoramic view of northern Marin County. It felt like a private club. There were no women present. The entrée was a boneless chicken breast stuffed with spinach, goat cheese, and caviar.

"Emilio," Storch said. "We'll have our coffee in the executive lounge, with some of the chef's special lemon soufflé to follow. Ask him to sprinkle on some of that old brandy he keeps in his desk." He turned to Gabe. "I hope you don't mind, old man. It's the only place they'll let me smoke."

They sat in leather armchairs, looking out over the Kimberley grounds. When the waiter went away, Gabe asked, "Why the move to Kimberley, anyway? I thought you were the rising star at Crystal Labs."

Storch lit a cigarette. "They were too damn tight with the pursestrings. I had this lovely new drug almost ready to start Phase Two trials and they were planning to sell it off because they couldn't afford to finish the testing."

"This is Virazine you're talking about?" Gabe said.

"Yes. They sent me out here to negotiate a deal with Ed. He suggested that I might want to come along as well."

"Whose idea was it to bring along your friends Howard and Sheila?"

Storch looked across at Gabe with a sheepish grin. "I keep forgetting. You're a reporter now." He tapped the ash off his cigarette. "My old bosses were a bit cross with me. But there's no point in breaking up a winning team. Not with a drug as promising as this one. Ed was most enthusiastic at first. Unfortunately, he has a short attention span. And he talks a better game than he plays."

"There were no problems with the testing?" Gabe said.

"Not that we know of. What have you turned up?"

Gabe hesitated. "Look, I promised Kate I'd only tell Arthur. Maybe you could arrange to sit in with us."

"Of course, old man, of course. I don't want to get you in trouble with your lady friend." He smiled. "You gave me quite a shock for a moment there, old man. But I really can't imagine that there's any kind of serious problem with Virazine. I think once you see our testing reports you'll agree. . . . Anyway, no use becoming upset before we have to, right? And certainly not before we've had our dessert."

21

"I should warn you not to take Arthur too seriously," Storch said, checking his reflection in the polished brass paneling of the elevator. "He's retiring soon. He'll be out of here in a matter of weeks." Storch made a face. "The sooner the better as far as I'm concerned. His replacement is already waiting in the wings."

McCauley's secretary was the friendly woman with the warm brown eyes and salt-and-pepper hair who'd been watching the gardening tape down in the gym. She looked up from her computer keyboard and took off her earphones as they came in.

"I feel I know you, Dr. Austin," she said. "I enjoy your column and your pieces on the news." Gabe couldn't help feeling he had seen her on TV, advising arthritis sufferers to take the headache remedy doctors recommend most.

"So is the good doctor ready for us?" Storch said.

"Yes. You can go right in."

Gabe followed Storch into the inner office. A short, stocky man with white hair, a white beard, and black hornrimmed glasses sat at a large mahogany desk making notes on a yellow legal pad. A pair of brass masks, one smiling, one frowning, hung on the wall behind him.

Storch cleared his throat. McCauley looked up at them, slightly startled.

"You're early." McCauley's mouth twisted in displeasure. Gabe glanced at his watch. They were right on time.

"Good afternoon, Arthur. This is Dr. Gabe Austin. Gabe, Dr. Arthur McCauley." Storch seemed a bit embarrassed.

"Yes, yes. The famous columnist and TV personality. At your service, Doctor. At your service." He rose, bowed, and waved them to a seat. "When any potential regulatory problem rears its ugly head behind these hallowed walls, you will inevitably hear the Kimberley Labs battle cry: 'Dust Off the Doc.' Well, sir, I am duly dusted. So, if you please, tell me what complications you plan to add to my last weeks in this august position."

"Arthur." Storch leaned forward in his chair. "Dr. Austin is here to tell us about a possible problem with Virazine."

"Ah. Is that so?" McCauley stared with mock gravity across his desk at Gabe. He used his eyebrows the way an orchestra conductor might use a baton. "Well. I have underestimated you, sir. I did not realize that you were a pharmacoepidemiologist as well as an all-around media celebrity. Please *do* tell me about your research."

Gabe did his best to ignore McCauley's condescending tone. "Three patients," he said, sliding the charts across McCauley's desk. "All taking Virazine. Malignant hypertension. Uncontrollable. I'll leave the conclusions up to you."

"How kind of you." McCauley straightened the files on his desk without looking at them. "We shall

159

look into them, of course," he said. "But, as I trust Dr. Storch has already told you, we didn't have any serious problems in our Phase Two and Phase Three testings. I suspect that these people died from something totally unrelated."

"You haven't received any other serious ADRs on this?" An ADR is an adverse-drug-reaction report.

"Absolutely not. Anything as important as this would have to be reported to the FDA, as I'm sure you are well aware."

"Arthur." Storch shook his head. "I think we need to take this very seriously."

"Quite right, sir. Quite right." He nodded gravely, turning to Gabe, the corners of his mouth turning up in a smile. "But do let me explain why I'm not planning to have an immediate cardiac arrest over your news." He folded his hands on top of the charts and looked at Gabe over the black rims of his glasses.

"Kimberley has nearly seven hundred pharmaceutical representatives in this country alone. Most U.S. physicians see one of our reps at least once a month. It's the most natural thing in the world for them to mention a questionable symptom in a patient taking one of our new drugs. I'm sure they would let us know if their patients experienced *any* ill effects."

"So you've had no reports on Virazine at all?"

"Oh, there may well be the odd case of diarrhea and perhaps a headache or two. But rest assured, we'll pass these on to the FDA as we're legally required to do."

"You can save yourself the trouble," Gabe said. "I Fed Exed copies to a friend at the FDA yesterday. I'll give you a week to look into it and get back to me."

Storch's face went pale. He clenched the arms of his chair. McCauley's face had turned a bright shade of red. He slapped his hand down on the charts. "Is that meant as a threat, Doctor?" he asked.

Gabe smiled. "Not at all. I've done you a favor by not going public already. I'm giving you a chance to do the noble thing."

"And after a week?"

"It depends on your response. I'd suggest you hold a press conference to announce what you've found. I don't need to be the one to break the story. But people deserve to know."

"Your arrogance surpasses all tolerance, Dr. Austin. You come waltzing in here trying to bait us with some cock-and-bull story about Virazine. You then announce that you've already blown the whistle to the FDA. Now you threaten to trumpet these slanderous allegations far and wide. Either you lack all sense of decency or you simply don't appreciate the problems your actions will produce for us."

Storch had recovered his composure. There was a sad, resigned expression in his eyes. He leaned forward and said gently, "Calm down, Arthur. After all, we should be grateful that Gabe brought this to us instead of putting it out over the airwaves."

"Perhaps you've forgotten, Dr. McCauley," Gabe said. "Physicians are strongly encouraged to report any questionable drug effects to the FDA."

McCauley looked as if he was about to come around the desk and attack Gabe physically. Storch rose and stepped in between them.

"Gentlemen," he said. "I think it might be wise to adjourn this meeting now. Gabe, I think you've done what you came to do?"

"Yes."

Storch nodded. Gabe saw the distress in his face. "I'll give you a call tomorrow to let you know what

161

we've come up with. I think that's the very least we can do, Arthur. Don't you agree?''

McCauley looked at Gabe as though he'd much prefer to be flayed alive. "We'll give it our full attention," he said. "But you'll have to forgive me for not being overwhelmed with gratitude. You of all people should know that anecdotal case reports are fiendishly difficult to substantiate—or to disprove." He nodded curtly and did not offer to shake hands.

As they went out, it seemed to Gabe that McCauley's secretary looked at him strangely. She appeared ready to say something, but at the last moment changed her mind. Gabe wondered if she had been listening in on their conversation and was angry at him for giving her boss a bad time.

22

Kate stepped out from behind her desk, straightening a stack of yellow pads in a wooden tray. "I just spoke with Ed," she said, looking up at him sharply. "I have to tell you, Gabe. I'm pretty upset."

"Yeah, I can see." News traveled fast. It couldn't have been more than half an hour since he and Storch had left McCauley's office. Storch had taken him back upstairs to apologize for Arthur's bad manners and to pledge his best efforts to resolve the problem.

He said he would put together an in-house task force to review the testing and postmarketing surveillance on Virazine, and that he personally, would fly down to San Diego to look into the two cases there. Storch said he would also call the company's sixteen district sales managers to ask them to be on the lookout for similar cases.

"So what did he tell you?" Gabe asked.

"He said you were down in Arthur McCauley's office, accusing us of faking the testing on Virazine." She was looking at him under lowered eyelids. Her jaw moved from side to side.

"Hey, hold on a second . . . I never said—"

"I also understand you've already reported your cases to the FDA. Is that true?"

"Listen. You're upset. Why don't we sit down and talk this over."

"I prefer to stand." She stood with her arms crossed over her chest. "Did you?"

Gabe shook his head, put his hands in his pockets, and paced to the other end of the room. "McCauley was acting like a total jerk," he said. "He implied that I was making a big stink out of nothing and that he was going to take his own sweet time investigating this thing. I got kind of steamed, sure."

"Did you really submit those cases to the FDA?"

He nodded. "I sent copies of the three medical records to Ken Weber."

"When?"

"I dropped them off at the Fed Ex box on the way to your place. Kate, I had a moral responsibility—"

"Don't give me that bullshit. You could have let us know first."

"Sure. And I could have forgotten all about Lindsey. I watched the pathologist slice up her brain like you'd slice up a loaf of bread—"

"Gabe—"

"—then I find two other patients taking Virazine who died of the same thing. So what the hell do you expect me to do? Sit on my hands?"

"You lied to me about the FDA. And you broke your promise." Her chin was shaking.

"You're right. I did," he said. "Because I was afraid my feelings for you would get in the way of my better judgment."

"You used me, you bastard. And to think I've been working my butt off to get Ed to offer you a job . . ." The tears were coming now. Gabe saw that some tender softness deep beneath her defenses had been exposed. A part of him wanted to stop this stupid argument, to shut his mouth and put his arms around her and tell her that everything would be all right. But, to his horror, he saw that it was already too late. She was advancing on him with an air of physical threat.

"You lied your way into my bed. You tricked me into bringing you up here. You have completely undermined my credibility as a professional woman. You had no right to take advantage of me—of our relationship—to get into Kimberley to drop your dirty little bombshell."

"Wake up, Kate," he said. "Talk about conflict of interest. Your whole fitness program depends on the success of that drug. You're promoting it, for Christ's sake."

"Gabe," she said, grasping one hand with the other, "I'm not denying the possibility that there could be a problem with the drug. I'm saying it's extremely unlikely. Yet you're ready to destroy a great medicine on the basis of what will almost certainly turn out to be a few chance occurrences."

"Okay, Kate. What's done is done. What do you want me to do now?"

"Let the company and the FDA carry out the investigation. Don't take it to the media until all the evidence is in. Your unsubstantiated headlines will be all over the front page. And when the drug *is* finally vindicated, it's a two-line story on page twenty-two. And the drug is dead. Forever."

"And Kimberley Labs loses millions of dollars. And your whole little fantasy of running a health spa out in the country goes up in smoke. But I don't suppose that has anything to do with it."

She picked up a copy of the *Physician's Desk Reference* and threw it at him. The book glanced off his shoulder and fell to the floor. "Damn you. Dean and I really stuck our necks out for you. Did you know that?"

"Yeah? And why was that?"

"We thought you could use the goddamn money. But you'd blow it all in a minute for a chance to make Ed Elias look like Adolf Hitler. You're really convinced Virazine is responsible for these deaths, aren't you?"

"If I had to go by my gut feeling right now, I'd have to say yes."

"I've had just about enough of you and your goddamn hunches." She pushed him toward the door. "You want a fight? You're going to get the fight of your career. Get the hell out of my office. And out of my life."

23

The lobby of the Kimberley Laboratories building was dim, cold, and quiet. Gabe was considering his alternatives when the elevator doors opened and Sheila stepped out. She was wearing a gray flannel jacket and skirt over an emerald green silk blouse. She slipped on a pair of dark glasses and hurried toward the door of the parking garage.

Gabe called to her. Sheila heard his voice and stopped suddenly. In her high heels she was nearly as tall as he was.

"Well. Dr. Austin. What a nice surprise." She did not look altogether pleased. She bit her lip, glancing around quickly. Her skin was pale and transparent, like one of those plastic anatomical models that show the vessels and organs beneath the skin. Gabe realized that she was not wearing makeup.

"No, stop," she said, taking a quick step backward, tottering unsteadily. "Don't come too close. I . . . I don't want you to catch my cold."

"Listen," he said. "I'm in a jam. Can I catch a ride back to Fairfax with you?"

Sheila looked confused. She hesitated.

"If it's a problem, I can call a cab," Gabe said.

"Oh no." She smiled. "No problem. Forgive me. I . . . I was up working all last night. Let me . . . just let me just pop into the ladies' room before we go."

As they walked to the garage she seemed quieter, more relaxed. Sheila's dark blue BMW looked like it had recently been through a car wash and had a fresh coat of wax, but the inside of the car was a jumble of newspapers, old fast-food wrappers, and stacks of forgotten file folders. The passenger seat was piled high with sets of self-improvement tapes in their big plastic packages: *How to Be the Person You Always Wanted to Be, Peak Performance,* and *Take Control of Your Time and Your Life.*

"Sorry for the mess." She dropped the tapes on top of the rubble in the backseat. As they neared the entrance of the parking garage, a car backed out in front of them and Sheila braked to a sudden stop. Another tape package came sliding up under his feet. Gabe picked it up. It was an eight-cassette package titled *The Psychology of Self-Esteem.*

"So tell me," he said. "What do you get from these things?"

"How to behave," she said. "How to think. How to act." Her voice was so soft he could hardly hear her.

"Why do you need a tape for that?"

"Your parents were obviously there for you when you were little."

"Yeah. I suppose." The bright flower beds flashed past outside his window.

"So there's a lot you take for granted. I didn't have that. I had to teach myself how to dress, how to talk, how to put on makeup. I didn't have the luxury of having a mother to teach me those things."

"Why not?"

"My family came apart. My brother and I were split up and shipped off to live with strangers." She shrugged. "I'm still trying to learn how to get it together so people will like me." She smiled and reached behind Gabe's seat to pick up a thin four-color catalog. "Speaking of which, here's something you might like," she said, dropping the catalog in his lap. "I wasn't sure I had any of these left."

It was a faded mail-order lingerie catalog. He looked across at her questioningly.

"See if you can find anybody you know in there," she said. Gabe found Sheila on page 6, wearing a black silk camisole and tap pants. She appeared a half dozen times throughout the catalog, each time wearing a different garment: a wine-red Victorian velvet robe, a black lace bra and panties, a pair of men's white silk pajamas, unbuttoned far enough to reveal most of one small pale breast, and something called a merry widow, all black sheer gauze with dangling garters. On one page she was pictured in a languorous cat-stretch, wearing a low-cut slip with a lattice of straps across the back. On another page, she was laughing, turning away from the man she was posing with, her leg up over his thigh. She appeared on the back cover in a demure blue-ruffled dress.

"Now you know how I worked my way through business school."

Gabe looked up from the photos to Sheila. Her eyes were red and puffy behind the dark glasses. In the harsh light of day she looked old, worn, and exhausted.

"Can I ask you a personal question?" she said, glancing over at him as she pulled onto southbound 101.

"Sure," he said.

"Will you to promise to tell me the truth?"

"All right. If you'll answer a question of mine."

"Truth or dare." She nodded, smiling. "I promise. You go first."

"What was it you took? In the washroom?"

"You bastard."

He waited.

"Here," she said. "You tell me." She fumbled in her purse and handed him a small folded Zip-Loc bag. Gabe shook half a dozen pills out into his hand. They were little purple football-shaped tablets.

"Xanax," he said. Xanax is an antianxiety medication, a member of the same drug family as Valium.

She nodded. "Like I said, I've had a couple of rough days. We've had some killer deadlines at work."

"What else?" Gabe said.

She gritted her teeth at him. Then she shrugged. "What the hell," she said. She dug another plastic bag from her coat pocket. This one contained tiny yellow tablets the size of a pencil eraser. There was a K inscribed on one side of the tablet. The other side bore the number 4. It was Dilaudid, a powerful and addictive narcotic.

"Where the hell did you get this?" he said.

She shook a long finger at him. "My turn." She smiled wickedly behind her sunglasses. "Do you really find Kate Reiley more attractive than me?"

"You really want to know? Even if it hurts?"

"Especially if it hurts," she said in a mocking voice.

He licked his lips. "You're a beautiful woman, Sheila. But you're too goddamn desperate. You give men too much power. The truth is, I'm more attracted to Kate."

She drove in silence, slumped over the wheel. All

the playfulness had gone out of her face. "And you wonder why I take Dilaudid," she said at last.

Marty Dorland sat with one foot up on a worn black ottoman. He was a huge unmade bed of a man. His desk was stacked high with review copies of books on cats, Hollywood personalities, the latest diets, pop psychology, cookbooks, and more cats. His wastebasket was overflowing with releases from every publicist west of the Mississippi. Marty, who suffered from gout, was an ex-restaurant critic with a drinking problem. Gabe sat across from him in his crowded cubicle at the *Chronicle* features department.

"Look. Gabe," he said in his gravelly voice, handing Gabe back his story. "Nothing personal, buddy, but there's no frigging way we can run this."

"Why not? You haven't even read it."

"I don't have to. It's about this new pill from Kimberley Labs, right?"

Gabe laughed, tossing the manuscript back across Dorland's desk. "No. It's about the common side effects of high blood pressure drugs."

"Really? That's funny. Don Kelsey from legal called up to tell me you were about to turn in some damn story that was going to get us sued. He got some kind of phone call about it. Earlier today."

"Oh yeah? From who?"

"I don't know. He said he'd heard you were out there stirring up trouble."

"That's my job, Marty. But I haven't written anything about it yet."

Marty shook his head. "Look Gabe, I'm sorry as hell, but stirring up trouble is *not* your job. Don tells me we're talking three-year legal action, minimum, okay? You got any idea what that would cost? Not to speak of losing a good advertiser. If you think there's a problem with some drug of theirs, do me a favor, take it up with the FDA. But don't write about it in my paper."

"Too bad Woodward and Bernstein didn't have you for their editor, Marty. Nixon would still be president."

Marty shrugged. "That's life, baby. I'm just trying to keep the features department out of trouble, okay?" He shook his head again and brought his feet to the floor. "This is a service piece, remember. You want investigative journalism, go call *60 Minutes*. Now, I got some ideas for next week: new ways to clean your teeth. Exciting. How to fight killer dandruff. Investigation at its best. Or you really want to be a prince, tell me three easy steps I can use to get rid of these goddamn hemorrhoids."

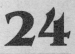

24

At 8:45 the next morning Gabe sat at a table at the Espresso Emporium, across the street from the offices of KSF-TV. He was drinking a *café latte* and looking through the TV Ideas file Lu Jean had prepared. The best of the lot was a piece copied from a drugstore trade magazine: "Child-proof Tops Foil Seniors." Elderly customers with arthritis were having trouble removing the child-proof caps from their medications. There was a handwritten note in Lu Jean's precise calligraphy:

A simple issue people can relate to. Great visuals. The Mt. Zion Elders Program would be glad to have you come shoot their daycare clients any weekday between 1 and 4 P.M. Call Gail Franklin, 863-3186. And let me know if you'd like me to round up a selection of bottles with child-proof caps.

—Lu Jean

Gabe put away the file and ordered a second *latte*. That should do it for this week's TV spot. He took out a yellow pad and began to brainstorm ways of turning the Virazine story into a TV piece.

At 9:25 he was in the KSF-TV control room watching Audrey Meyers, the producer/director of *Wake Up, San Francisco*. She sat at a high desk wearing a headset with an attached microphone, looking down over a row of light, sound, and video control boards to a wall of TV monitors. An earnest student intern, a slight, dark woman with a boy's haircut, hovered at her side.

"Camera three, that's too wide," Audrey was saying. "Come down a little. I'm getting glare at the top of the picture. Yes, that's better. Ten seconds. Penny, cue Jim to speed it up. We're almost out of time. Hurry up, Jim. That's it. Penny, tell him to cut it quick. Beautiful. Okay, Charlie, go to the commercial. Good. Okay. Whew! Super. We're out of here."

Audrey bounced up out of her chair and began throwing scripts, pens, and papers into her oversized briefcase. "Great work, team. You guys are the great-cst. Scc you tomorrow. Jcnnifcr, you can takc a break now, dear. I need to go talk with Dr. Austin."

She turned to Gabe. "Good morning. Walk with me, will you? We're going upstairs."

She led him down a long carpeted hallway that led from the studios to the front of the building. Gabe hurried along, half a step behind. Audrey had always intimidated the hell out of him.

"Wally Pinkwater woke me up at six this morning," she said, stopping on a quiet landing halfway up the stairwell. Pinkwater was the station's vice president for sales and marketing. "Can you picture that? Wally Pinkwater calling *me?* At home? He must have yelled at me for ten minutes." Audrey and Pinkwater were not on the best of terms. He had been lobbying the general manager to replace half an hour of her show with reruns of Oprah Winfrey.

"Why?" Gabe said. "What happened?"

"One of our big advertisers called him. Kimberley Labs."

"I didn't know Kimberley was an advertiser."

She nodded grimly. "Flea collars," she said. "And Wally knows the president out there, what's his name . . ."

"Ed Elias."

"Yes. Wally's apparently been sucking up to old Ed for years." She started up the stairs again, motioning impatiently for him to follow. "And now it's beginning to pay off. Their flea collars are doing great and they're about to launch a new line of over-the-counter medicines or something. When they do, there'll be this monster ad campaign." She seized his arm, pulling him to a stop outside Pinkwater's office door. "Before we go in, tell me quickly—what's the story?"

"Well, Kimberley Labs has this very promising new drug that helps cure herpes."

"So they want you to give it some coverage? Yeah, I see the problem. Herpes is such old news. . . ."

"No, that's not it," Gabe said. "The drug has a bad side effect. It raises blood pressure. I think it may have killed some people. They want me to keep quiet about it."

She waggled a finger against his chest. "So they're worried you're going on my show and tell our viewers this big bad drug company is trying to slip this potentially dangerous drug over on them so they can make a fast buck? Am I right?"

"Yeah, that's basically it."

"And are you?"

Gabe shrugged. "I've reported it to the company. I've reported it to the FDA. If they all sit on it, and we find some more cases, I might propose—"

"Wrong." She put a hand flat on his chest. "Look, darling. Here's how it works: The people who hire and fire around this station are the people who sell the ads. It's that simple. You piss off our advertisers, you're history. You're a real talent. I'm talking maybe network someday, if that's what you want. But I could have a pretty good new TV doc in here before lunch. And Wally could get a new producer/director just as fast."

Gabe nodded. "I get the picture."

"I hope you do. Because I happen to like this job. Now I'm going to go in and tell Wally this is all a big misunderstanding. We have no plans for any such story. We haven't talked about it. You haven't proposed it. We're not going to do it. Period. Now I can do that *with* you or *without* you. So what'll it be? You want to come tell him yourself or do I go in and tell him you just resigned?"

25

Gabe set his alarm for 4:30 A.M. and called Ken Weber at home. Weber was a clinical pharmacologist who had trained in Gertrude's lab. He had gone on to become one of the country's leading pharmacoepidemiologists. He now worked at the FDA.

"Yeah, I got your charts," Weber said. He did not sound enthusiastic. Gabe could hear children's voices in the background. "You come up with any other complicating factors?"

"No. Have you received any other adverse reports on Virazine?" Gabe asked.

Weber hesitated. He sounded troubled. "They would normally go to the company first. You checked with them?"

"Yeah. They think I'm making it all up."

"It's going to be hard to get a lot of action right now," Weber said. "You know we got a new head of PMS last month?" PMS is the FDA's division of postmarketing surveillance.

"I heard there was going to be a shakeup," Gabe said. "Who is it?"

"Milton Stonecipher."

"Stonecipher. Jesus. I thought he was the number-two guy in Infectious Disease."

"He was. I take it you've had dealings with Uncle Miltie before." The nickname was ironic. Stone-cipher was among the least avuncular of men.

"I've written him and tried to call him a dozen times," Gabe said. "He's always put me off to someone else."

"Uncle Miltie's gotten himself pretty well invested in Virazine. He's the one who fast-tracked it through when he was running Infectious Disease. Something bad happens, his ass is going to be in a sling. You're going to have to hit him with a whole boxcar of hard evidence before he'll take any action on this sucker."

"So why is he so hot for this drug?"

"Politics. We've been under a lot of pressure to speed up approval on all the antivirals and all the AIDS drugs. Virazine is both. You know they're using it to treat cytomegalovirus now?" Cytomegalovirus infections of the brain are common in advanced cases of AIDS.

"Yeah. So I've heard," Gabe said.

"So there's really not a hell of a lot I can do from this end," Weber said. "I'm two levels down from Stonecipher and the division heads have absolute discretion on these kinds of things. Send me anything else you come up with and I'll make sure it gets on his desk. But I sure as hell wouldn't hold my breath."

"I haven't hit a ball since my college days, you know," Gabe said.

Storch pulled their golf cart up to the driving range. He was wearing a plaid golf cap and windbreaker and matching bright blue trousers. Gabe wondered why it was that men would wear clothes on a golf course they wouldn't be caught dead in at home. He had worn a sweatshirt, jeans, and an old pair of Nike trainers.

They hit a few balls and Storch handed him a red plastic stadium cup.

"What's this?"

"Joseph never could learn to make a decent frozen margarita." Storch poured his cup full of ice-cold lime-green slush from a stainless steel Thermos. "I finally had to buy the club a machine—in exchange for a free lifetime supply. You have to help me recoup my investment."

A round of golf had been the last thing on Gabe's mind. The interview with Pinkwater, KSF's vice president for sales and marketing, had been humiliating. Kate had not returned his calls. He had been planning to indulge himself with his all-time favorite bike ride down on the Monterey peninsula. But Storch had been so sympathetic about the flap with Kimberley, and there had been such a desperate undertone in his voice, that Gabe had decided to change his plans and drive up to San Rafael that afternoon.

They had met in the little bar at the Kimberley Creek Golf Club, the company's golf course. Storch had waved away all his attempts to talk about business. "Later, old man. Let's get out to the first tee."

Gabe didn't have his own set of clubs and was forced to ask the pro shop for a rental set. After a hurried search the attendant had located a dirty green bag of scarred metal clubs and had strapped it onto the back of their golf cart next to Storch's custom-made bag.

"I'm surprised you want to be seen with me," Gabe said as they got into the cart. "I seem to be *persona non grata* around the company."

Storch chuckled. "I don't let Ed Elias do *all* my thinking for me."

Gabe leaned back in his seat, sipping his drink. "It's cold," he said.

Storch nodded. "You have to take it slowly or it'll give you a hell of a headache. Shall we?"

Storch drove the cart across a wooden bridge to the first tee. He took his driver out of his bag and looked down the fairway. "Shall we say a hundred dollars? I'll spot you ten strokes."

Gabe laughed. "Come on, Dean. I haven't played in a dozen years. How about ten dollars and twenty strokes?"

Storch gave him a exasperated look. "All right, all right. Twenty dollars and fifteen strokes then. You won't get an offer like that every day."

"How did Ed take it?" Gabe asked, as he joined Storch at the first tee. "The Virazine business I mean."

"Not too well. Ed has too much invested in Virazine to want to hear any bad news at this point." Storch shrugged. "I told him we should try to work with you, not against you. Pool our information. Personally, I believe that you've acted very honorably. Would you like to lead off?"

Gabe took a few practice swings, reminded himself to keep his eye on the ball, and hit it a hundred yards up the left side of the fairway. His ball rolled up to the top of a little knoll on the edge of the rough.

"Not a bad start, old man." Storch teed up, took two easy practice swings, and hit his ball a hundred seventy-five yards down the middle of the fairway.

"Somebody is really putting on the pressure," Gabe said as they got back into the cart. "There've been calls to the *Chronicle* and KSF, trying to shut me up."

Storch nodded. "I'm afraid Ed has sicced Ray Brody on you."

"Ray Brody? What's he got to do with this?"

"He came by yesterday after you left. He and Ed

had a long chat. I got the idea Ed had asked him . . ."

"Asked him to what?"

"You know. Try to work something out."

Gabe felt a dark, sinking feeling pass down his backbone. "I hear that anybody Brody considers too inflexible could be facing a radical change in his life expectancy."

"That was the old days, old man. Ray has pretty much gone legit these days. Of course, his old contacts do come in handy every once in a while."

Storch hit a long approach shot that rolled onto the green. Gabe dribbled his way toward the pin with a 7 iron.

"Look, Gabe. I know Ray," Storch said, pulling his putter from the bag. "He's not an unreasonable guy. He's smart, he's creative, and he's a great deal maker. He might be able to help us work this out. I'd rather deal with him than Ed any day."

On the next hole Gabe sliced his drive far to the right. He finally found it under an inch of water. As he was trying to decide whether to wade in and play it, Storch came down the bank, scooped out the ball, and threw it back onto the fairway. "California rules," he said.

As they got back into the cart Gabe said, "By the way, what's the chance of getting copies of your pre-marketing testing on Virazine?"

Storch shook his head. "Personally, I'd be delighted. But I'd have to get Arthur or Ed to approve its release. And I don't think they'd do that for you right now." He waited to let another cart cross a bridge over a small creek. "On the other hand, it's very convincing stuff and I'd love to have you see it. Tell you what. Come on up to my house and I'll let you look through my own copy. I've been wanting to show you my new place anyway."

Storch won their wager by a dozen strokes. But he refused to take Gabe's money. He insisted on driving them up to his house in his sleek green Jaguar.

"It's only a mile and a half, old man. Nothing at all. I'll drop you back at your car."

He pulled out of the club, lighting a cigarette from the car lighter. He noticed Gabe's discomfort and rolled down his window, letting the light mist blow in on the shoulder of his golf jacket. His face was soft with alcohol and unaccustomed companionship.

Gabe had worried about Storch's driving after all he'd had to drink, but the man piloted the sleek Jaguar sedan flawlessly. Even so, Gabe breathed a sigh of relief as they turned off the freeway at Lucas Valley Road.

They passed through a residential neighborhood and came out into open country. The road narrowed and became crooked and steep. Gabe caught glimpses of black and white Holsteins standing in hilly pastures. Five miles up the road, Storch pulled in at a private gate and punched at the electronic keypad mounted on a metal post. The gate opened and they drove on up the hill.

"The executive vice president of Transamerica lives right over there," Storch said. "The villa across the way belongs to the family that owns the Giants."

"Fat City," Gabe said.

Storch gave him a modest, slightly embarrassed shrug. They continued for another mile up the twisting, narrow private road. Gabe rolled down his window. He could smell the bay laurel.

It was a wooden Japanese-style house on top of a hill. Storch drove up the steep driveway past an elaborate walled garden. The door of the three-car garage swung up as they approached.

"Nice place."

Storch nodded, gesturing absently at the house and grounds.

"This was my big project when I moved out here," he said. "I'd been doing a lot of traveling to Japan. The temples and the architecture really made an impression on me. I only come up on weekends now. Ed built us all these darling little condos on the company campus. I usually stay there during the week."

"You still getting up with the owls?"

"Oh yes. I try to get to my desk by five or five-thirty. It's the only time I get any work done." He pulled in beside a red Porsche convertible and led Gabe into a big, bright, bare room next to the garage. There were half-a-dozen skylights. A row of high windows ran across one wall. A row of narrow glass doors looked out onto the garden. An empty easel stood in the middle of the room.

"The painting studio, old man," Storch said, his voice heavy with irony. "You can see how much I get to use it."

Gabe shook his head. "I couldn't imagine you ever wanting to give it up."

"Perhaps I'm fooling myself, but I like to tell myself I'm saving it."

"Saving it?" Gabe said. "For what?"

"For when I retire." Storch smiled, shrugged, and crossed the room to open the French doors.

Outside, a wide deck overlooked a formal Japanese garden with an elaborate artificial streambed. At the lower end of the garden was a large pond covered with water lilies. Several massive boulders stood in the midst of raked sand.

"Come on, Dean. How old are you now? Fifty? Fifty-two?"

"I'll be fifty-eight in another month."

"You don't have to retire. You could just could come up here and paint. It's like one of those temple gardens in Japan."

"It's modeled after one of them," Storch said. He flipped a switch beside the door. Water began to flow down the artificial streambed. A wave of water washed down the face of a boulder beside the pond.

"Excuse me for a minute, will you?" Storch said. "I need to make a quick call. Help yourself to anything you like at the bar." He went back inside through the French doors.

Gabriel walked toward the pond, trying to imagine what it would be like to live in such a place. A dozen large, blood-red fish moved in the black water.

A few minutes later a screen door closed and Storch emerged from the house with a worried smile.

"I just spoke with Brian. He's Ray Brody's nurse. He said Ray is up and around. He'll try to bring him over in about twenty minutes."

Gabe was irritated. "Dean," he said. "What the hell?"

Storch lit a cigarette, put the lighter on the table beside him, and blew smoke up into the dark sky. "Ray lives right down the road. He hasn't been well lately. We're all pretty sure he has AIDS, but he keeps denying it. So we don't talk about it anymore. He's had full-time care for the last year, big clean-cut muscular young men. Over these last few months Brian has become his butler, his chauffeur, his major domo, his bodyguard, and who knows what else. Anyway, what can it hurt? Unofficially. Just the three of us. Maybe we can work something out. If not, we're no worse off than before. Would you like to look over the Virazine test results until he gets here?''

Storch set him up at the desk in the study. Gabe settled himself and began to read through the research reports. It was deadly dull. After fifteen minutes he went to the sound system to put on some music. He found a tape in the player—cassette 4 of *The Psychology of Self-Esteem*.

It was more than an hour later when Storch knocked on the study door.

"They're here," he said.

It was raining lightly now. Gabe and Storch stood under the covered part of the deck and watched the white Rolls limousine come creeping up the steep driveway. The driver, a massive, blond weight-lifter type, came around to the back door and gave Brody his arm. They made their way up the walk, Brody walking stiffly with the help of a heavy ivory cane, the younger man holding a large black umbrella.

Ray Brody was an emaciated man of sixty, short and grave, wearing a finely tailored trench coat over a three-piece suit. He had heavy-lidded eyes and a weathered complexion that spoke of a lifetime of regular trips to Palm Springs, Acapulco, or Hawaii. Storch introduced them.

"A pleasure, Dr. Austin," Brody said. There was a blazing intensity in his eyes. His hand was small, dry, and strong. He had a strong Boston accent.

"And this is Brian."

"Hello, Brian." Gabe saw that he was very young. He also seemed uncertain. He kept glancing over at Storch as if for cues.

"Dr. Austin. Good to meet you, sir." Brian got Brody settled in his chair.

"Mr. Brody. I've heard a lot about you," Gabe said.

"Likewise, Doctor. Likewise. All of it perfectly flattering, I'm sure. Sit down, sit down. Brian, you can make me my usual, if you would."

"Sure thing, Mr. Brody."

"What I was hoping we could do here, Ray, is what you're so good at," Storch said. "Focusing in on each party's interests and trying to work out an arrangement that gives everybody what they want."

"The professor here is such a nice boy, isn't he," Brody said to Gabe. "Wouldn't hurt a fly. He's so goddamn sweet and earnest people don't notice how crafty and slick he really is." He turned to Storch. "What do you want to be so goddamn nice for, Dean? I thought Ed wanted us to scare the shit out of him."

"This is my party, Ray," Storch said. "Let's play it my way."

"Whatever you say, Professor. Be nice now. We can always scare the shit out of him later."

"You'll have to forgive this guy, Gabe. He grew up on the streets and never learned to behave."

"Just the opposite, Professor," Brody said. "I like to think of myself as a kind of Miss Manners of the business world, you know? I try to teach people to behave in a civilized manner. You take a nice idealistic young fellow like the doc here. He's not a bad guy, he's just getting himself into unknown territory. He hasn't learned the behavior code. Or the dress code either, from the looks of it."

"Give us a break, Ray." Storch smiled. "We were out playing golf."

"No kidding. I thought you'd been to your mother's funeral." Brody tossed down the last of his drink. "I'm going to bury you in that damn jacket."

"Ray, we're here to consider *everybody's* interest," Storch said. "Now as I see it, Gabe's main interest, as a journalist, is to be the one who breaks this story. He doesn't want to get scooped. That's a very reasonable request and I think we could guarantee that, maybe even arrange for him to break it on national television. I believe you know the producer of the *Today* show pretty well. Am I right?"

Brody smiled modestly, raising his hands, palms up, in a dismissive gesture.

Gabe felt the blood rise in his face. "I don't believe this," he said. "You think I care about that? My 'interest' is in keeping people from dying. I thought we were coming up here to pool information so we could try to figure this thing out."

"What did I tell you," Brody said. "A bleeding heart all the way."

"Shut up, Ray," Storch said. "Gabe, I'm for that too. What do you want? I'll tell you anything you want to know."

"Fine," Gabe said. "Has the company received any more ADRs on Virazine?"

"No," Storch said. "I checked. Not a one."

"That's odd," Gabe said.

Storch shrugged. "How about you? What have you and Gertrude figured out so far?"

Gabe leaned forward in his chair. "We're looking at four possibilities," he said. "Number one: we're dealing with a straightforward MAO inhibitor reaction. The drug is directly responsible for the deaths. But there's something about the victims that makes them especially susceptible."

"You figured out what that might be?" Brody asked.

Gabe shook his head. "Number two is a two-drug interaction. Virazine interacts with something else. Call it Factor X."

"Okay," Storch said. "What else?"

"Number three: Virazine has nothing to do with it," Gabe said. "It's some outside agent, something else entirely. An especially virulent strain of herpes. Another drug. Some kind of environmental toxin. We're calling that Factor Y."

"I vote for that one," Storch said.

"Gertrude and I have already started some lab work," Gabe said. "Trying to figure out the mechanism."

"How are you doing that?" Brody asked.

"We're trying to create an animal model."

Brody looked blank.

"They're giving Virazine to a bunch of rats," Storch said. "Then exposing them to various other substances."

Brody made a face. "Sounds like a real blast."

"Ray doesn't like rats," Storch said.

"You said there were four possibilities," Brody said.

"Yes. Number four is a contaminant," Gabe said. "The drug itself is fine, but something nasty got into the vat. That's what's causing all the problems. We need you to track that one down for us. Did all the victims get Virazine from the same batch?"

"I'll check that out for you," Storch said. He took out his pocket notebook and made a note.

"I see what you mean, Dean," Brody said. "You're a nice guy, Doc. A hell of a nice guy. You kind of vindicate my faith in human nature or something." He turned to Gabe. "So, down to business. What do you think of this consulting job?"

"I think that's rather a moot point just now, don't you?" Gabe looked to Storch. "I mean, do you really think . . ."

Storch shrugged. "Business is business, old man. Ed may be a bit anxious about Virazine right now, but his long-term intentions haven't changed. Our offer is still open."

"Let's talk about that later," Gabe said.

Brody frowned. "Is it the money you're unhappy with? We might be able to—"

"It's not the money," Gabe said.

"Good," Brody said, taking an envelope from his breast pocket. "This will be an advance payment for your first five days as a consultant."

"It's not the money," Gabe said. He did not take the envelope. "It's the muzzle."

"The what?" Brody said, cupping a hand behind his ear.

"The muzzle," Storch said. "He thinks we want to put a muzzle on him."

"A muzzle." Brody smiled as if he liked the idea. "No, no. Nothing like that. You needn't worry about signing the contract until we've dealt with the whole Virazine matter."

Storch nodded. "We don't intend to pressure you, Gabe. And we'd never presume to advise you in matters of journalistic ethics."

"That's right," Brody said, picking up the envelope. "Ed would like you to take this check simply as a sign of his goodwill. You don't even have to cash it until this whole business blows over. If you change your mind and want to give the money back, you can do so at any time."

"So I'm free to do what I want about breaking this story?"

Brody shrugged. "If you want to go public with this, how can we stop you? We're just asking you to do us this little favor: wait for a few days. I understand you haven't even had a chance to read over the original premarketing testing."

"I was just looking at it inside. It's going to take

several days to get through it. And I'd like to have Gertrude Potter take a look at it too."

"I'll tell you what," Storch said. "You agree to hold off on any publicity for the time being and I'll have a complete set of the test results in Gertrude's office by noon tomorrow."

"You've got a deal," Gabe said. "We'll hold off at least until we've had a chance to look over the tests. After that, it's going to be a judgment call."

"By that time, I hope we'll have new evidence that will show that this is all just a terrible misunderstanding," Storch said.

Gabe nodded. "Good luck."

Brody smiled as if Gabe's comment had been addressed to him. "My luck is generally quite good," he said, heaving himself up out of the chair as Brian hurried over to take his arm. "I'll just leave this with your friend Dr. Storch." He handed Dean the envelope. "And, Doctor? Please stay in touch. We don't want anybody to do anything they might regret."

Gabe and Storch stood on the deck and watched the big car roll slowly down the hill.

"You see?" Storch said. "He wasn't so bad."

"Bad enough," Gabe said.

"You're sure you don't want this?" Storch said, peeking into the envelope. "Twenty-five big ones. You don't get handed one of these every day."

"I can't take it, Dean."

"Of course you can, old man."

"No."

"All right, then. I'll hold on to it for you." He put the envelope in his breast pocket. "By the way, have you spoken with your friend Dr. Jefferson lately?"

"Michael? Not since I was in San Diego. Why?"

"He's come up with another of his computer-matched cases. A woman who works in a dry cleaning shop.''

"Yeah?" Gabe felt his stomach tighten.

"Yes. I called down there yesterday. He was going on and on about that medical diagnosis program of his. It really sounds quite fascinating. I promised to put him in touch with a San Diego investment banker I know.''

"Let me guess," Gabe said. "You just happened to dangle some venture capital money and Michael just happened to spill his guts on this new case he'd found.''

"Not at all, old man. He specifically asked me to pass this information on to you.''

Gabe swallowed his irritation. "So what happened?" he said. "This new case—was she taking Virazine?''

"No," Storch said. "That's the interesting thing. There's no evidence she'd had any contact whatsoever with the drug. No evidence of herpes either. Yet, she had the whole range of symptoms you've described.''

"Did she die?''

"No," Storch said. "She pulled out of it. We've asked Dr. Jefferson to look into some of the cleaning solvents she'd worked with. Ed feels that it may be an important new lead.''

26

Gabe's plane arrived in San Diego at 10:05 the next morning. Michael Jefferson was waiting for him just past the taxi stand, sitting at the wheel of his red Porsche convertible, reading a copy of *Omni*. He saw Gabe, waved, and got out of the car.

"Hey, buddy." He took Gabe's bag, patting him on the shoulder. "You still mad or what?"

Gabe gave Michael's hand a perfunctory shake. "Jesus, Michael. What do you think?"

"Look, man, I'm sorry. I really am."

Gabe let out a long breath. "It was a little weird to hear about the new case from Dean Storch. What the hell's going on?"

"I didn't call him, man. He called me. He said you were all working on it together, and he'd be glad to pass on the details. I never thought it would be a problem . . ." Michael opened the trunk and put Gabe's bag inside.

"Yeah, okay," Gabe said. "I'm sure you had other things on your mind."

"Damn right." Michael's eyes sparkled. "Guess who I just did a demo of the system for?"

"Who?"

"AT&T. Can you believe it? A-fucking-T & T."

"That's great. I'm happy for you, Michael." Gabe managed a grin. "So—did you rent me a car?"

"Hey, man. I thought I'd just loan you mine."

"Your Porsche? You're kidding."

"Little peace offering," Michael said. "You can drop me off at the hospital on your way."

"I'll take it, I'll take it," Gabe said. He opened the door and slid behind the wheel. The leather seat was soft and cool against his back.

"Can't have my main man mad at me, now can I?" Jefferson got in on the passenger's side.

"Forget it," Gabe said, peering down at the controls. "Tell me about your Mrs. Davis."

"Fifty-six-year-old black lady," Jefferson said. "Came to the ER on Monday afternoon complaining of dizziness and a headache."

"Uh-huh," Gabe said. He started the engine, waited for a break in traffic, and pulled the car gingerly away from the curb.

"Her pressure was sky high. Didn't respond to Hyperstat. The whole bit. You want to stay in the left lane here. The freeway entrance is the next block on your left."

The little car was surprisingly responsive. Gabe felt the wind in his hair. "But she didn't die," he said.

"No, she pulled out of it," Michael said. "She works at a dry cleaner's. I was thinking it might be some kind of chemical exposure. It's all in here." He tapped the manila envelope in his lap.

Gabe pulled onto the freeway. Traffic was light. When he stepped on the gas the acceleration threw them both back against their seats.

"You're sure she wasn't taking Virazine?"

Michael shook his head. "Negative. I asked her myself," he said. "But you said you wanted to hear about *anybody*."

"Sure. What else can you tell me about her?"

Michael bent down out of the wind to read the chart as Gabe drove toward the ocean. Mrs. Davis's pressure was 195 over 143 when she went to the hospital. It had gotten as high as 215 over 162 and did not respond to the usual treatments. Over a period of five hours her pressure gradually returned to normal.

"It's like she got a lighter dose of the same medicine," Gabe said. "Any others?"

"Negative," Michael said. "And I've run a search every day. There's the hospital. You can turn in right here."

Gabe shook his head. "Doesn't exactly sound like an epidemic, does it?"

He pulled over to the curb in front of the emergency entrance. Michael paused, his hand on the door. "What did your friend Elias have to say?" he asked.

"They don't believe a word of it," Gabe said. "He thinks it's all some plot to make the company look bad. You sure you want me to take this buggy down to south San Diego?"

"Hey. No problem," Michael said, getting out and closing the door behind him. "It's insured."

The W. W. Wright Drive-In Cleaners on West Parker Drive had originally been a gas station. The high facade was now painted in bright red and yellow stripes. A large plastic sign admonished passersby to Stay Stylish the Wright Way. There was a cartoon of a middle-aged gentleman with a big smile, a bald head, and a bow tie.

A bell tinkled as Gabe went in. The room was deserted. A display of leaflets on the counter offered tips on cleaning everything from afghans to zoot suits. Plastic-draped clothing on hangers hung from a motorized rack that angled down from the high ceiling. The plastic rippled in the breeze of a large industrial fan.

A cheery young woman came out through a swinging door and raised her eyebrows. She looked like a high school cheerleader on her way to a pep rally.

"Something to pick up, sir?"

Gabe shook his head. "I'd like to speak with Hattie Mae Davis, please."

"I'm sorry sir. The workers in back aren't permitted to have visitors."

Gabe frowned. "I'm Dr. Austin from the University Hospital. It's important."

She took a step back toward the door. She seemed to be inspecting his necktie. "I'd better let you talk to the manager," she said.

She went back through the swinging door. A few moments later a sunburned young man in a red jacket, red tie, and yellow shirt took her place, glancing over Gabe's shoulder at the Porsche. He looked as if he had been practicing his smile in front of a mirror. His name tag identified him as Trevor Pruet.

"Yes, sir. How can I help you today?"

"I'm Dr. Austin from the University Hospital in San Francisco." He handed Pruet a copy of his business card that identified him as a fellow in Gertrude's lab. "I need to see Mrs. Hattie Mae Davis."

"Nice of you to come check on her, Doc, but she seems just fine today. No problems at all." The cheerleader came out behind him and leaned against the wall.

"I'm glad to hear it," Gabe said. "But I still need to see her. Several other patients have come down with similar symptoms. It appears that there may be some kind of an epidemic. I need to ask her a few—"

"I don't know that I can do that, sir. If I pull her off the line it's going to shut down our cleaning process for a while. We've got a big backlog to get out by six and I'm not authorized to pay any overtime. Is there any other way I can help?" His smile grew even tighter. It looked to Gabe as if it was putting a considerable strain on his face.

Gabe did his best to look puzzled. "Gee, Mr. Wright was very concerned that we get our investigation over with as soon as possible. I guess I'll have to ask him to give you permission. Mind if I use your phone?"

Pruet swallowed hard. "Oh, well, if Mr. Wright . . . You wait right here, Doctor. I'll see if I can't figure out some way to spring her loose for a couple of minutes."

He disappeared into the back. A Vietnamese youth in a red T-shirt came in with a tangled pile of shirts and trousers. A few minutes later a soft-faced black woman in a yellow uniform peered out through the glass of the swinging door.

"Are you Mrs. Davis?"

"I sure am. You the doctor who wanted to see me?"

The cheerleader gave Gabe a disapproving look. "Why don't you two go on back?" she said. "The floor workers aren't supposed to be out here."

Gabe made his way through the swinging door into a small hallway beside a wheeled rack of freshly ironed shirts. It was noticeably warmer here. Mrs. Davis squinted up at him uneasily. "I don't believe I recognize you, Doctor."

"No, ma'am. We've never met. I'd like to ask you about the problem that brought you to the emergency room on Monday. We've had several other people with the same symptoms and we . . ."

She kept looking back over her shoulder. "I'd like to help you out, Doctor, but I really don't know that I can take the time right now. This here Mr. Pruet is new on the job and he's going to get himself in trouble sure. I feel fine now, I really do. Maybe I could come talk to you on my lunch break."

"All right," Gabe said. "What time do you get off?"

"I can trade with Mary Beth and take my lunch at eleven-thirty."

"Okay. I'll be waiting out front in a red car. I'll take you to lunch."

Mrs. Davis came out at at 11:35. Her eyes widened when she saw the Porsche. Gabe reached across the passenger seat and opened the door for her.

"My goodness. I never been in one of *these* things before," she said, her eyes sparkling. "It's so low. How do you get in?"

Gabe got out and went around to help her in.

"Wait till I tell my nephews about *this!*"

She directed him to a Mexican coffeeshop a few blocks up the street. He led her to a quiet booth in the far back. She ordered a hamburger and a Pepsi. Gabe had tortilla soup and iced tea.

"Are you back to normal now?" he asked.

"Yes, sir. I believe so, God willing. I hope the Lord Jesus don't see fit to make me go through anything like *that* again."

"How did it start?"

"Well, sir, I'd just got off work. My sister picked me up and carried me over to her house. Her husband, Rupert, just got promoted to chief mechanic down at Southport Toyota. She was putting on a spaghetti dinner for some of his friends. It wasn't till after dinner that I took sick." Mrs. Davis took a bite of her burger. She had already finished her packet of potato chips.

"What was the first thing you noticed?"

"My head. It started hurting like crazy. I couldn't hardly see. I had to lie down on the sofa it hurt so bad. Finally my brother-in-law, bless his heart, he stopped the party and took me down to the emergency room."

"What happened when you got there?"

"All these doctors swarmed over me. Kind of scared me. They put needles in my arms, bright lights in my eyes. There was this band they wrapped around my arm that they kept inflating. There must have been a dozen doctors running around. You never saw anything like it.

"And when I started to feel better, they asked me all *kinds* of questions about the dry cleaning shop, the chemicals and all. They even called my boss, Mr. Wright, and him practically an invalid after his heart attack and all." She let out a muffled snort. "I told them, they the same chemicals we been using for fifteen years."

"Had you been sick in the last couple of months?"

"No, sir. Nothing to speak of."

"Anything at all?"

"No, sir. As far as I know, I've always been healthy as a horse."

"Not taking any medications?"

"No, sir. I never took nothing else but what they give me down to the hospital."

Gabe lowered his voice. "You'll have to excuse me, Mrs. Davis. Some of the questions I have to ask are a little personal."

"That's okay, Doctor. I understand."

"Have you had any venereal diseases in the last

few months? Any rashes or sores in your genital area?"

"No, sir. Nothing like that. But come to think of it, you know what I did have?"

"What?"

"The chicken pops. Just a couple of weeks back. I caught it from my little niece. She brung 'em home from kindergarten. I don't know *why* I never got it when I was a baby like everybody else. I had to stay in bed for three or four days. I had it bad. I was itchy all over and I had all these little red bumps just like they say."

"Did you take anything for it?"

"My sister did give me a couple of leftover pills my niece was taking when she had it."

"Do you remember the name of the drug?"

"No, sir. I sure don't."

"Do you still have the container the pills came in?"

"My sister maybe does. I can give you her number."

Mrs. Davis's sister, Emma Tucker, was cool but polite on the telephone. She didn't remember what the chicken pox medicine was called, but she thought she still had the bottle around somewhere. She said Gabe was welcome to come by and she'd see if she could find it.

The Tuckers lived on the second floor of a municipal apartment complex fifteen minutes away. The outside of the building was filthy and the parking lot was littered and unkept. Gabe locked the car and turned on the security alarm.

Mrs. Tucker was a calm, dignified woman in a white dress. Her apartment was scrupulously tidy. "I still haven't found the medicine you wanted, and I've been through the whole cabinet. There's just a couple more drawers I still have to check."

Gabe helped her look. They found the empty bottle in the back of a bathroom drawer. The prescription had been written for the son of one of Mr. Tucker's fellow mechanics. The label read:

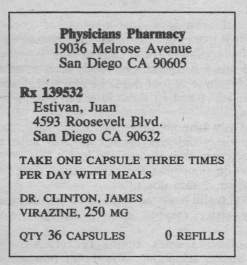

Physicians Pharmacy
19036 Melrose Avenue
San Diego CA 90605

Rx 139532
Estivan, Juan
4593 Roosevelt Blvd.
San Diego CA 90632

TAKE ONE CAPSULE THREE TIMES
PER DAY WITH MEALS

DR. CLINTON, JAMES
VIRAZINE, 250 MG

QTY 36 CAPSULES   0 REFILLS

27

It was long after midnight when Gabe let himself into his apartment. Michael had taken him for an early dinner at a French restaurant in San Diego and they had put away two bottles of an excellent red wine. The dark weight of a headache pounded behind his eyes.

The lock on his front door would not respond to his key. It was some time before he realized that it was unlocked. His first thought was that Lu Jean had forgotten to lock up. When he opened the door he smelled the lingering traces of cigarette smoke.

There was a dark shape on the floor next to his feet. Gabe nudged it with his toe. The bundle emitted a low wail.

Gabe flipped on the overhead light. Someone had put Princess in one of the pillowcases from his bed. The open end of the pillowcase had been closed off with a rubber band. Gabe felt his muscles tighten. He took a deep breath, blowing it out through his mouth. He removed the rubber band from the pillowcase. The cat emerged from the sack and ran to hide behind the couch.

He checked the other rooms. Someone had been through the papers in his office. He looked through his files. As far as he could tell, nothing was missing. There was no sign that anyone had gotten into the pharmacy, either. On an impulse, he emptied the trash can under the sink. At the very bottom, wrapped in a paper towel, he found three crushed cigarette butts. Vantage Filters.

Gabe coaxed the cat out from behind the couch and held her on his lap until they had both calmed down. He moved to the end of the couch and dialed a familiar number. His uncle answered on the second ring.

"Uncle Larry? Sorry to wake you. This is Gabe. Somebody broke into my place. I wanted to make sure you were okay."

"Yeah, I'm fine." His uncle's voice was thick with sleep. "Broke into your apartment?"

"Yes. Nothing missing."

"Did you check the store?"

"Yeah. Nobody's been in there. You notice anything unusual before you left?"

"No. How did they get past the alarm?"

"Beats me. I just wanted to make sure you were all right. We'll figure it out in the morning."

Gabe was out of cat food so he gave Princess a can of tuna. She sniffed at it suspiciously, looking up at him as if to ask whether there was some mistake. While she was eating he went into his office to listen to his phone messages.

"Hey, Gabe. This is your man in Washington. Good news, bad news, buddy: Don't quote me on this, but the rumor is Uncle Miltie's planning to leave FDA. That's the good news. Here's the bad news: He's slated to become the new medical director at a certain Marin County drug company. Over and out."

"Dr. Austin, this is Betty in Dr. Crowell's office at St. Catherine's. We've got you down for a thirty-six-hour shift beginning Friday night at eleven. Please call to confirm. Thanks very much."

"I've got a message here for Dr. Gabriel Austin," said a deep male voice. " 'Free legal advice, Doc. I think you should take a nice vacation. You're a nice guy, Doc. Nobody wants to see you get hurt. But you're up against some big, bad people here.' That's the message." Gabe played the message back again, copying down the text. After listening to it a third time, he was fairly sure that the caller was Brian, Brody's nurse-bodyguard.

"Gabe? Are you there?" It was Sheila's voice. She sounded half-drunk. "I've been thinking of you, you sweet man. I found out something you need to know. Give me a call when you get in. No matter *how* late it is. *Ciao* for now."

Gabe reset the tape, got a cold bottle of Grolsch from the refrigerator, and took his pile of medical journals back to the living room couch. He called Kate's number, got her answering machine, and hung up without leaving a message.

He missed Kate so much he could hardly stand it and he was afraid of calling Sheila when he was feeling so vulnerable. He opened the big bay window and sprawled on the couch, looking out at the sign across the street: 4 HOUR SPECIAL SERVICE.

Sheila, Sheila. What am I going to do with you? he asked himself. *Come on. Admit it,* he told himself. *You enjoy her sexy little games. Those little touches on the arm. Those quick glimpses down her blouse. All that seductive little-girl bullshit.*

He put on his coat, went downstairs, and walked east on Clayton Street, passing the good cheap French restaurant, the Chinese food place, and the pizza delivery outlet. At the health club on the corner he crossed the street and walked down to the Tassajara Bakery, looking in the window at the spotless floors, the bentwood chairs upside down on the round tables.

He walked back along the other side of the street, past the Vietnamese vegetable market, the hardware and video stores, the cleaners, and the foreign-car garage. He stood in front of the wine shop and looked up at his own bright open window across the street. *Okay,* he told himself. *Time to shape up. If she's found something, I need to know.*

He crossed back to his side of the street and read the menu in the window of the Ironwood Café. The dining room was empty, the floors freshly scrubbed, the chairs stacked on the bare tables. He pictured himself coming here with Kate. She would order the mussels marinara and he would have the grilled salmon with the sorrel cream sauce. They would split a good bottle of chardonnay. From a long way off he smelled the breeze from the ocean.

"Gabe. How nice of you to call."

"Hello, Sheila. How're you doing?"

"Oh, not so good."

"You drinking?"

"You can't ask that," she said.

"I'm asking."

"Will you come over and see me tonight?"

"No can do, kiddo."

"Gabe. I really need you. Please say you'll come."

"You sound scared."

"I am."

"What about?"

"I . . . I can't tell you."

"Why don't you come over for breakfast," he said.

"I'm really afraid I won't make it through the night."

"I'll meet you at the emergency room at Marin General."

"No . . ." There was a long silence. "Why is it that when I'm with you, I feel I can let that wall down and just be a goddamn little girl again?" she said.

"I don't know, Sheila," he said. "Maybe it's because I don't want anything from you."

There was another long silence. "I guess I find that pretty hard to take," she said at last. He heard the cars going by outside in the rain.

"Gabe?" She sounded hopeless and lost. "Why don't you like me?"

"I like you fine, Sheila. You give me too much power, that's all. Come to breakfast at seven. I'll make you some yogurt pancakes."

"All right," she said. "I'll be there. And, Gabe? Thanks. Nobody else talks to me the way you do. See you in the morning."

Gabe tossed the journals to the floor and put his feet up on the couch. He heard the clang of the cat door and Princess came in. She jumped up beside him and pressed her head against his midriff. He scratched behind her ears. She purred louder, pressed herself against his leg, and tried to stand on her head.

28

Sheila stood in his doorway grinning madly, clutching a bundle of yellow roses. She took off her coat, shook out her hair, and stepped up and kissed him.

"So this is where you live," she said.

"This is where." He had already broken a half dozen eggs into a big mixing bowl. She rummaged in his cupboard for a vase.

"I find that when I'm feeling bad, it cheers me up to buy flowers. Do you ever do anything nutty like that?"

"Sure. I tend to buy bicycles, though."

"Yes. So I see. Mind if I use your bathroom?"

"Not if you're planning to take any drugs."

"Just a pee, darling. Honestly. Just a pee."

She came out a few minutes later, fresh and composed. "You don't mind if I take a look around your apartment, do you?" she asked. "I'm so curious about how you live and work."

Gabe shrugged. "Go ahead. Take a look," he said. "It's not much."

Gabe heard her humming to herself in the other room. He was relieved to have her out from underfoot. He prepared the batter, cooked the pancakes, put them in a hot oven, squeezed the orange juice, and set the table. When everything was ready he went down the hall to call her to breakfast.

Sheila was sitting at his desk, leafing through a stack of papers. The patches of light and shadow moved on her face as if some tiny creatures were crawling beneath her skin. He realized that what he was seeing was simply the motion of her jaw. She was chewing gum.

He felt a flash of anger. "Sheila. What the hell?"

"Oh, Gabe. I'm . . . I'm sorry." She recoiled, pushing the papers away from her. "I was . . . I was just looking . . ."

"Looking for what? It looks like you're ransacking my goddamn office."

She looked up at him like a cornered rabbit. "I'm sorry," she said. "I didn't mean to pry."

Gabe hesitated. "Well, breakfast is ready. I guess we might as well eat."

"Yes," she said. "Let's eat." She attempted a smile. "I'll be good. I certainly didn't mean to be pawing through your things."

Sheila finished her breakfast, put down her fork, and reached across the table, linking her fingers in his, looking at him pensively. "You sure don't look like the enemy," she said.

"How's that?"

"Ed's been issuing bulletins inside the company. He seems terrified that you're going to blow Virazine out of the water. He says we've got to do everything we can to stop you."

Gabe warmed up their coffees. "He's doing pretty damn well so far," he said.

"I heard them talking about some guy named Santini," she said. "Does that name mean anything to you?"

"Santini? No. Should it?"

"I . . . I may be totally off the wall, but I have an idea this Santini is some . . . well, I don't know. I shouldn't . . ."

"Come on, Sheila. Who is he?"

"I might be wrong, but I got the feeling he was some kind of tough guy from out of town. Somebody they're bringing in to scare you or shut you up. I've never seen them like this."

"Why are you telling me this?"

She took his hand and brought it to her cheek, shaking her head and smiling a winsome, contented smile.

"Oh, I don't know," she said. "Maybe it's your eyes. I've always been a sucker for strong, gentle men with pretty blue eyes. No, you stay still. You're going to sit there and drink your coffee while I clean up."

Two hours later Gabe stepped out of the elevator and into Gertrude Potter's lab. A young Asian man was transferring a series of Erlenmeyer flasks from a metal cart into a big refrigerator. A tall, bearded student was working at a computer keyboard. A chinless young woman stood at a high lab bench, catching the drips from a glass column in a test tube. She told Gabe he would find Dr. Potter down in the animal room.

He rode the elevator down and found Gertrude standing at a high table, inspecting an anesthetized white rat under a binocular viewing scope. Gabe wrinkled his nose at the smell.

"Oh, Gabe. Hello. Will you help me? I am so frustrated today. I need to measure the size of the tumor on this poor mousie, but I cannot see the numbers on the measuring screen."

"Let me take a look." Gabe looked through the scope. The rat's abdomen had been shaved. In the middle of the bald area was what appeared to be a darkly pigmented small black mole. He adjusted the measuring grid. "I'd say it was about four millimeters by six millimeters."

"Thank you. It makes me so mad when my eyes don't work." She bent over the table to write in her black lab notebook. She finished writing and closed the book. "How good to see you. Here, help me sit down."

Gabe helped her lower herself onto the high stool. She reached out to pat his arm. "I am getting too old. Too old," she said, smiling up at him.

"You're going to outlive all of us and you know it."

"It is not so bad to die, you know. Americans are not so fond of dying. But it can be quite a good thing. Just think. No taxes to pay. No more dishes to wash. No more being nice to the chairman of your department."

"Gertrude, Kate was telling me you helped develop the nerve gas derivative for Kimberley's flea collars."

"Oh, yes. I got to work with Howard Pearlman. He's a very nice boy. Very bright."

"How long have you been working for Kimberley?"

"Well of course I knew Dean at Yale. I did some consulting work for him when he was at Crystal Labs. These drug companies pay very well, unlike some academic institutions." She paused. "He just sent me a big box with all the original test results on Virazine."

"Yeah? What do you think?"

"They did a good job of testing for MAO inhibitor

activity, so they may have had some reason to think there might be a problem. But I can assure you, they didn't find it," Gertrude said. "The tests were all negative. Every one. And there's no way they could have fudged the evidence on this one."

"So much for that," Gabe said. "Did you get Lindsey's lab test back?"

"Yes. It was positive for MAO inhibitor activity."

Gabe nodded. "I was pretty sure it would be. So where do we go from here?"

"We try to see what other things these patients of yours have in common. We try to figure out the mechanism. And we do some testing to tell us if our guesses are correct."

"These people at Kimberley and the FDA are going to keep stonewalling until we can come up with an ironclad explanation of exactly what's happening and why. But that could take months."

"Not necessarily," Gertrude said. "There is much we can learn from our mousies, if we only know how to ask."

29

Steve Duncan, chief of the Department of Radiology at San Francisco General Hospital, was a lean, brisk, balding man with scraggly blond ringlets. He wore a long white coat over bleached blue jeans and a cranberry silk cowboy shirt. Gabe found him sitting in front of a mechanical viewing screen, talking into a dictation phone, a half-eaten box of jelly doughnuts and a Thermos of coffee on the desk beside him.

"Well. The half-court reprobate. We've missed you on Saturdays," he said, reaching up to shake Gabe's hand. Steve and Gabe were regulars at the weekly pickup basketball game at the UCSF gym.

"Things have been crazy lately," Gabe said. "Look, Steve. I've got a problem."

"Come on back." Duncan picked up the box of doughnuts and headed down the corridor, motioning for Gabe to follow. His office was small and tidy. Duncan closed the door.

"I've got a series of three ER deaths," Gabe said. "Hypertensive blowouts. One of them was Alex Troutman's daughter."

Duncan nodded grimly. "I heard. What a tragedy, huh. Any leads?"

"They were all taking Virazine."

"The new herpes drug?" Duncan let out a low whistle.

"I've got two identical cases and a near miss in San Diego," Gabe said. "Kimberley is denying there's a problem. They're doing everything they can to shut me up."

"Can't say I'm surprised." Duncan refilled his coffee and reached for a doughnut. "What can I do to help?"

"I was hoping you might let me have a peek into your patient database."

"Looking for?"

"Death from hypertensive crisis in patients on Virazine."

Duncan shook his head. "Sorry, buddy. No can do."

Gabe's shoulders slumped. "You're kidding," he said.

"Nope. Definitely against hospital policy. I could really get my ass in a sling."

"Great, just great. How would you suggest—"

Duncan held up a hand. "I have now officially said no to your request. But now I'm aware there might be a problem. As a responsible physician, what do I do?"

Forty-five minutes and four doughnuts later, Duncan looked up from his keyboard. "Looks like we've had six deaths among all our people taking Virazine," he said, tapping his computer screen with a fingernail. "That's awfully damn high, considering our doctors have only written a hundred and two scripts for the stuff in the four weeks it's been on the market. Let me break them out by chief complaint."

A moment later the printer began to clatter. Duncan tore off the printout and they looked at it together.

Patient	Age	Admitted for	Received Virazine for
Baker, Gladys	72	Cataract surgery	Herpes simplex keratitis
Hernandez, Carlos	34	AIDS	CMV infection
Lee, Ching Ma	54	Malaria	Genital herpes
Lindenbaum, Richard	49	AIDS	CMV infection
McMillan, Walter	74	CA of bladder	Varicella
Valman, Robert	43	AIDS	CMV infection

"Three of the six had AIDS," Gabe said.

"Throw those out and you've still got three deaths out of a hundred scripts. Not very good odds."

"Don't throw them out yet," Gabe said. "Can you get cause of death on this thing?"

"Sure." Duncan pressed a succession of keys. There was a long pause. A new list came up on the screen.

Patient	Age	Cause of Death
Baker, Gladys	72	Hypertensive crisis
Hernandez, Carlos	34	Cerebral aneurysm
Lee, Ching Ma	54	Cerebrovascular accident
Lindenbaum, Richard	49	Klebsiella pneumonia
McMillan, Walter	74	Hypertensive crisis
Valman, Robert	43	CMV infection

"Right on the money, ace," Duncan said. "Four out of six could have been the result of elevated blood pressure."

"But was their pressure up before they died?"

"You'd have to look in the charts for that," Duncan said. "I'll get you copies by tomorrow."

"Get me two of each and I'll Fed Ex a set to Ken Weber at FDA."

"Great. I'd appreciate that," Duncan said. "Getting something Fed Exed out of here is like building the pyramids. I'll notify Sol Thomas. I'd better call Bill Goldman as well." Thomas was the hospital's chief of medicine. Goldman was San Francisco's director of public health.

"Maybe this'll be enough to get the media interested," Gabe said. "Mind if I use your phone?"

It took Gabe twenty minutes and considerable verbal horsepower to get Stu Zolar on the line. The KSF news director was not a man to beat around the bush.

"Okay, Doc, what have you got for me?" he said. "It better be good if you want to get it on tonight's news. We've got a press conference at the mayor's office and a big protest over at the navy shipyard."

"How about a drug scandal featuring a local manufacturer?" Gabe said. "I've got seven suspicious deaths in patients taking Virazine."

"What the hell is Virazine?"

"Kimberley Labs' new antiherpes drug. It appears to have some kind of rare but lethal side effect."

"Any of the deaths in the city?"

"Four at General, one at St. Kate's."

"You're sure you can back this one up, Doc?" Zolar said. "I can't afford to let you shoot from the hip like you did with that eggplant-diet scam."

"Trust me, Stu. I'm over at General now. I'll get copies of the charts. I've got photos of some of the victims. I'll have a statement from one of the docs over here."

"Okay. Sounds like we'd better take a look. Come by at two and we'll go over the story. Do I need to send a camera crew out to Kimberley for some B-roll?"

"I could shoot it from Kimberley headquarters." Gabe said. "Think about it. I'll be in your office at two."

30

So what are you telling me, Stu?" Gabe asked. "You just called Elias cold and he agreed to go on camera?"

"It was just a formality," Zolar said. "A courtesy thing, trying to be evenhanded. I didn't even expect him to take my call. We didn't think there was a chance in hell . . ."

They were standing in the back row of the Kimberley auditorium. A single cameraman adjusted his tripod on a platform in the third row. A man on a tall ladder was adjusting the stage lights.

"But he went for it," Gabe said.

"Yeah." Zolar shrugged. "Surprised the hell out of me."

"Maybe he's got some bombshell ready to drop," Gabe said.

"Maybe. There was one weird request. He wanted a table for eight of his top executives onstage."

"Moral support?"

"I don't think so. He's got something else up his sleeve. You all set with your opening statement?"

"All set," Gabe said. "Let me just read it through a couple more times before we get started." He took his script to a seat in the front row. He was able to read through it twice before the assistant producer snatched it out of his hands.

Sheila was showing people to their places at the long table. As Gabe watched, Storch, Kate, McCauley, and several others took their seats. Kate did not look at Gabe. Storch got up from the table and came hurrying down the aisle, leaning down to shake Gabe's hand. He seemed mildly amused.

"Give 'em hell, old man," he said. "I do feel a bit caught in between on this one. But I wish you luck."

"So Kate's going to be part of the show?"

"It's Ed's party. We're just minor players in this little drama." Storch looked down at the floor, as if seeking to spare Gabe the humiliation of witnessing the pained look on his face.

Elias appeared a few minutes before the taping was due to start. Sheila was at his shoulder. Elias looked down at Gabe, a grim expression on his face.

"Just couldn't contain yourself, hey Austin?" he said in a low voice. "Your big shot at bringing down a major drug company. You're making a big mistake. But I daresay you'll figure that out for yourself soon enough."

"Yeah, well, good luck to you too, Ed. Break a leg."

Sheila lingered behind and looked across at Gabe, confusion and concern on her face. Gabe gave her a smile and a thumbs-up gesture. She mouthed the words "good luck" and followed Elias away.

The assistant producer came to escort him to the stage. Gabe, Elias, and Brodner—the FDA spokesman—did microphone checks. Everyone was courteous and the run-through went smoothly. Gabe had to admit it was a class act.

As he took his place at the podium, the cameraman signaled three minutes. Gabe put in his plastic earpiece that let him hear Zolar's instructions. He glanced at the opening words on his script one last time, cleared his throat, and took a sip of water.

Staring straight into the camera, Gabe began, "Two weeks ago today, Lindsey Troutman died at St. Catherine's Hospital in San Francisco. She was seventeen years old. Until that day, except for a case of mononucleosis, she had been perfectly healthy. But because she had mono, Lindsey was given a new antiherpes drug called Virazine, manufactured here at Kimberley Laboratories in San Rafael.

"Since Lindsey's death, Channel Seven's investigative reporters have uncovered six more Virazine-related deaths, two in San Diego and four right here in San Francisco.

"Kimberley Labs has unofficially promoted Virazine as a cure for a wide variety of conditions caused by herpes viruses—genital herpes, cold sores, shingles, infectious mononucleosis, chicken pox, and the potentially fatal cytomegalovirus, a common complication of AIDS.

"But, for reasons that no one yet understands, some individuals taking Virazine appear to experience massive increases in blood pressure, often starting with a severe headache, and frequently ending in a fatal stroke or in other medical complications. Yet, the company insists that its drug is not to blame.

"Here with me at Kimberley headquarters is Kimberley's president, Edmund Elias. Mr. Elias, does Virazine pose a threat to the health of the American people?"

Elias, looking calm and controlled, turned to face the camera.

"Dr. Austin, these are very serious allegations. If there were a real problem with Virazine, you can be assured that Kimberley would be the first to sound the alarm. However, this drug has been tested more thoroughly than any other medication in history and has one of the safest side-effect profiles in the pharmaceutical industry.

"As you said, Virazine helps the body fight herpes. In fact, it's the most effective antiherpes drug currently available. Now, I can understand your own personal feelings. The young woman you referred to was a friend of yours. But I want to assure you—and the public—that any connection to Virazine was purely coincidental. This is a safe and very beneficial drug that will help save thousands of lives.

"We've thoroughly investigated the two San Diego cases you identified. Only one of those patients had received a prescription for Virazine. As for the patients at San Francisco General Hospital, these were very sick people, many of them with AIDS or other advanced diseases. These people died *in spite of* the drug, not because of it.

"To prove our faith in the drug's safety, I have asked several of my colleagues to join me in taking the maximum recommended dose of Virazine right now. As you watch. On camera. Ladies and gentlemen? Will you join me? If we could get a close shot of this . . ."

The camera zoomed in on the executives at the table. Sheila had passed out eight saucers, each one bearing three Virazine capsules. Kate, Elias, Sheila, and the others dutifully placed the capsules in their mouths and swallowed them.

"And so you see the level of confidence we at Kimberley have in this quality product. We are cooperating fully with the FDA and we are confident that further investigations will reconfirm what we already know: Virazine is a safe and effective aid in the battle against herpes."

Gabe cleared his throat and took his place at the podium. "Thank you, Mr. Elias," he said. "And now we have a response by FDA regional director Victor Brodner. Mr. Brodner, your response to the statements you've just heard?"

Brodner was a thick-necked bureaucrat of indeterminate middle age. He came blinking into the stage lights, looking down suspiciously at the microphone.

"Gentlemen," he said. "I can only say that this drug is in full compliance with all existing FDA regulations. It passed through its prerelease testing with flying colors. The cases you've mentioned have been submitted to the appropriate office in Washington and a full investigation is under way. FDA will give the matter a thorough review and will move with all possible speed to inform the public of our conclusion."

"Mr. Brodner, one last question," Gabe said. "How would you advise a friend or family member who was currently taking Virazine?"

Brodner looked evenly across the stage at Gabe.

"No one should stop taking Virazine on his own. The drug's benefits are well documented, while any allegation of risk is purely speculative at this time. Pending an official recommendation, I could only advise your viewers to check with their own physicians."

31

Gabe stepped out of the elevator in the Kimberly parking garage and walked toward his car. Elias had done a credible job, but he was satisfied that he too had done well. He had used a phone behind the stage to call the Associated Press to make sure they watched the piece. If they got it on the wire, it would be in tomorrow's papers across the country. Whatever happened, Kimberley would no longer be able to keep the controversy out of the news. And the FDA would be forced to give the drug an intensive review.

As Gabe was getting in he heard heavy footsteps running toward him. Instinctively, he locked the doors. A tall, bearded man in a brown jacket came running up to the car.

"Hey, relax, buddy. It's just me." It was Harry Blake, the sound man.

Gabe felt the tension go out of his shoulders.

He rolled down his window. "Hi, Harry. What is it?"

"A message from Stu. He wants to know if you wouldn't mind stopping back at his office for some kind of quick strategy meeting."

"A strategy meeting? Now?" Gabe had been hoping to catch a few hours of sleep before starting his hospital shift.

"I think you need to go, man. Old Stu sounded pretty worked up." Blake hesitated. "Hey, Gabe?"

"Yeah?"

"You were right-on tonight, buddy. Hang in there. These drug company people talk tough. But they've got to be running scared."

Gabe found Stu Zolar sitting alone in his dark office, looking out the windows at the lights of the Embarcadero.

"Stu?" Gabe hesitated at the door. "What's this about a meeting?"

"Just you and me, buddy," Zolar said. He turned his chair to face the door. There was restrained fury in his voice.

"What's the matter?"

Zolar shook his head in wry resignation. "I've just been on the phone with the general manager. He's going to get back to me about running the Kimberley clip."

"What?"

Zolar nodded. He was doing his best to be consoling. "The GM said you talked with Wally Pinkwater a couple of days ago about the possibility of doing a feature piece on Virazine."

Gabe nodded. "I was going to propose it as a feature on the Wake Up show. But Audrey Meyers shot it down."

Zolar chewed at his lower lip. "Wally was under

the impression that you'd agreed not to do *any* piece about Kimberley Labs. He passed that assurance on to the company. But that's neither here nor there. What bothers me is the precedent we're setting. We have a well-documented news story and by God—"

His telephone rang. He picked it up, said, "Zolar," into the mouthpiece, and listened, his eyes widening. As Gabe watched, the news director's face went white. He put his hand to his forehead and swiveled his chair away. He asked a few brief questions, then hung up the phone. He turned slowly in his chair and looked across his desk at Gabe, a silent accusation on his face. Gabe felt the blood rising in his cheeks.

"Ah, buddy," Zolar said. "I sure didn't want to have to hear that."

"What was it?"

"I wish to hell I could tell you. This is really going to tie my hands." He came around the desk and put a hand on Gabe's arm. At first Gabe took it as a sign of comfort. Then he realized that Zolar was attempting to get him moving out of the office.

"Stu. What the hell?" Gabe said.

"What can I say? When you're down, they kick you. When you're hurt, they kick you some more."

"Who was it? What did they say?"

Zolar stopped at the door of his office, shaking his head. "Someone from legal," he said. "I swear to God, Gabe. That's all I can tell you."

"But what the hell does it mean? Come on, Stu. Talk to me."

"I can't, buddy. I can't."

"So what are you telling me? You're definitely not going to run the piece?"

"Not tonight. Probably not ever. We'll be having

a board meeting in the morning. I swear to God I hope this blows over and you come out of it all right. But this is way out of my bailiwick. It's all up to the general manager now.''

Gabe pulled into the doctors' parking lot at the hospital at 11:45 that evening. A city ambulance was just pulling away. A van from one of the commercial transport services was idling in front of the ER door, its red taillights making a soft red glow under the heavy cement canopy.

Sandy, the ward secretary, was at her desk, filling out a long, imposing set of insurance forms. She looked up in surprise.

"Dr. Austin." Gabe saw panic in her eyes. She glanced away quickly "I . . . wasn't expecting you."

"No? I'm on the schedule. My regular weekend . . ."

"I . . . I'm not sure that you are. We tried to call you." She looked around desperately for help. Gabe turned to find Cliff Leslie standing there in a fresh white jacket, an ophthalmoscope in his hand. Gabe could tell from his face that something was wrong.

"Cliff. What are you doing here? I thought I was on tonight."

"I guess he didn't reach you, huh?" He shifted from foot to foot, giving Gabe a distant, embarrassed smile.

"Who didn't reach me?"

"Come in here. We need to talk."

Cliff closed the staff room door behind them. "It's Crowell. He's on some kind of a rampage. He called me this afternoon to say he'd taken you off the schedule and asked me to take your place."

"Unbelievable. Did he say why?"

Cliff shook his head. "No. But he's upstairs, waiting to see you. He said if you came in to send you up."

Gabe walked up the four flights of stairs as slowly as he could. He was certain that Ed Elias—or more likely Ray Brody—had gotten to Sid Crowell, perhaps under the guise of future funding for Crowell's research.

He found Crowell at his desk reading a medical journal.

"Well, hello. Come in, Austin. Have a seat." Crowell picked up his pipe and settled it between his teeth. It seemed to Gabe that he was trying hard not to look too pleased.

"Sid. What the hell's happening?"

"My office received an anonymous phone tip this morning. The caller said that a search of your locker would turn up something very interesting." Crowell cleared his throat.

"Yeah? So?"

"I had hospital security go down and take a look. They found a large quantity of Dilaudid. Nearly four hundred doses. We've determined that they're the same boxes that were taken from central supply last Thursday."

Gabe felt the anger rising inside him. So, it had come to this. They had set up some bullshit drug charge, an accusation that would never be proved, would never come to trial. But one that might destroy his public credibility.

"Come on, Sid," he said. "I haven't been anywhere near this place since my last shift. And you know it. You can open those damn lockers with a paper clip."

Crowell appeared not to hear. "The board has asked me to give you an opportunity to offer your resignation."

"Go to hell. The pills were planted."

"I will duly inform the board of your response. In the meantime, they have voted to relieve you of your duties, pending a full hearing."

"Great. And when will that be?"

"That's completely up to you."

"What do you mean?"

Crowell cleared his throat again. "You have a choice. You could have a public hearing. Charges would be brought and you'd have a chance to respond. The news media would be invited. You'd be entitled to bring your attorney."

"Great. What's my other option?"

Crowell pointed the stem of his pipe across the desk. "You can resign immediately. There would be no publicity, no formal charges. The whole matter would be dropped."

"Come on, Sid. That's blackmail."

"It's very lenient, if you ask me. You have some very solid supporters on the board, if I may say so. We all realize that you've been under a lot of pressure lately. There may be extenuating circumstances."

"And if I don't resign?"

"We announce your suspension immediately and hold a public hearing early next week. If the charges are confirmed, the board could either dismiss you from the staff or could negotiate some program of rehabilitation. Or we could opt to turn the whole matter over to the police."

"You've thought of everything."

"If you should wish to avail yourself of any of the hospital's psychiatric services, they would be provided gratis."

"How generous."

"The board has authorized me to keep our offer

open for forty-eight hours. I'm sure you'll want to seek professional counsel. And I would request that any communications with board members should go through me."

Crowell stood up. "I'm sorry about this, Austin," he said. His face was flushed with poorly concealed triumph. "You're a good doctor, and I know you mean well. It's always a shame when these things happen. I hope you'll be kind enough to call me day after tomorrow with your decision."

32

Gabe sat at his desk with his face in his hands. His whole life seemed to be crumbling under him. Kate hadn't answered her phone or returned his messages. He had passed up a very attractive consulting offer and had lost two of his three jobs. And, if he could believe Sheila, there was some muscle guy after him. All because he had insisted on running this Virazine business to the ground.

To hell with it. I've talked to the company. I've told the FDA. There's only so far a man can be expected to go. Maybe it's time to run up the white flag.

He turned to his bulletin board and looked at the photos of the victims. Juan Rodriguez smiled shyly from under the brim of his red baseball cap. Robert and Amy Blumberg stood in front of their new house, looking proud and prosperous. Hattie Mae Davis squinted into the sun in her yellow uniform. And Lindsey looked out at him, breathtakingly poignant in a recent cast photo. He had received two photos from the families of the patients at San Francisco General as well: Gladys Baker was a warm, motherly woman with her hair in a bun; Carlos Hernandez was a lean, handsome man with deep-set eyes and a Zapata mustache.

He pushed the button on his machine and sat back in his chair to listen. The messages were unremarkable except the first, from Sandy at the ER, telling him he was off the ER schedule, and the last two:

"Hello, Dr. Austin. This is Monica Penny. I'm a field producer for *60 Minutes*. Your letter has been forwarded to me. I'd like to fly out right away to do a preliminary interview. I'm at JFK now. I'll be leaving New York in half an hour. I'll phone you as soon as I arrive."

The last message had come in several hours later: "Dr. Austin, This is Monica Penny again. It's ten-thirty P.M. I've just arrived at SFO. I'll be staying at the Clift Hotel. I should be there in about an hour. Please call me there the *moment* you get this message."

Gabe called her room. Monica Penny answered on the second ring.

"Great. I was beginning to think you might be out of town. I'm exhausted. It's four A.M. for me. But we love your story idea and I want to talk to you first thing in the morning. The hotel dining room opens at seven A.M. If you could meet me then we could do a preliminary interview and I could go back and present it to my producer tomorrow afternoon. If everything works out, this could all be on the air this coming Sunday."

Monica Penny was a slim, elegant African-American woman in a teal suit. She rose to meet Gabe, extending a surprisingly large, strong hand.

"There you are. Right on time. I like that in a doctor." She wore tiny bright stars in her ears. They stood out against the dark chocolate-plum of her complexion like planets in the evening sky. She had an intense physical immediacy about her. Gabe guessed that she worked out every day.

"Shall we go on in? It's ten o'clock my time. I could eat a horse."

The maître d' greeted her like an old friend. He led them to a large, bright table in a rear alcove. She took her seat, shook out her napkin, and positioned a small black videocam on a tiny tripod on the table beside her, leaning over to squint into the range finder.

"That's it?" Gabe said. It looked like a child's toy. Gabe saw his reflection in the lens.

"That's it," she said, pushing a switch. A red light came on. "Sound and everything. Not broadcast quality, but damn close." She leaned across and put a hand on his arm. "So tell me more about this drug of yours," she said.

Gabe started with Lindsey and took her quickly through the sequence of clinical findings, pausing briefly as the waiter came and went. When he finished, she asked, "So what did the guy from the FDA have to say?"

"He waffled with distinction," Gabe said. "He looked with responsible concern at all sides of the question." He shook his head bitterly. "Getting a straight statement out of the FDA is like getting the Pope to chant 'Hare Krishna.' "

Monica tapped her gold mechanical pencil on the small yellow pad at her side. "Is it true that this drug was thoroughly tested and received a clean bill of health before it was introduced?"

Gabe nodded emphatically. "Yes. That's what makes it such a puzzle."

"How can you possibly explain that?"

"We think the drug is reacting with some new agent that wasn't around when the original tests were done."

The waiter brought their plates. She had ordered French toast with a double order of Canadian bacon. Gabe had asked for oatmeal and a bowl of fresh raspberries.

"Some new agent," she repeated. "Like what, for instance?"

"Some Substance X that reacts with Virazine to cause the problem," Gabe said. "It's got to be something that wasn't around when they tested the drug a year ago."

She shook her head, her fork poised in midair. "I don't get it."

"Something that wasn't in the environment at the time," Gabe said. "It could be almost anything: a new drug, a new virus, a new vitamin, a new environmental toxin, like a pesticide or a food additive. That's why it's such a puzzle."

"Sounds like a long shot. Besides, you've got what? Seven cases out of hundreds of thousands of people taking the drug?"

"Seven that I've found so far," Gabe said. "And one close call."

"But it could be a coincidence. The drug might not be the problem."

"There's always that possibility," Gabe said. "I'm not discounting it."

"Fair enough," Monica said. "So, say it *is* a new virus or whatever. How would that work?" She sliced a small triangle of bacon and stacked it on top of a perfectly square section of French toast. She speared it with her fork, mopped it in syrup, and popped it into her mouth.

Gabe took out a pen and a three-by-five card. "Let's say Virazine is normally broken down into two innocuous by-products," he said. He drew two benign-looking spheres on the card, labeling them A and B. "So they do the testing. And there's no problem."

"Okay," she said, "I'm with you so far."

"They finish the testing. Six months later, someone introduces a new cold remedy. It's a big hit. But one of the ingredients triggers an increase in the production of certain enzymes in the liver."

"Okay."

"With the increase in enzymes, Virazine is broken down into two entirely *different* by-products," Gabe said. He drew a triangle and a star, labeled them C and D, and underlined the star.

"It's one of these new breakdown products that produces the fatal reaction."

"Right, the MAO thing you mentioned." Monica raised her hand for more coffee. When the waiter went away, she asked, "Have you found any similar deaths among people who were not taking the drug?"

"No."

"What about the person who had the reaction but didn't die?"

"Yes." He told her about Hattie Davis.

"And you think she survived because she only took a few pills?"

Gabe nodded. "She only took two."

"Who else have you been working with to track this down?"

"Well, there's Michael Jefferson, chief of emergency medicine at the University of California–San Diego. Gertrude Potter, head of the pharmacology research lab at UC–San Francisco School of Pharmacy. And Steve Duncan, head of radiology at San Francisco General."

"And they'd be willing to verify your account of the deaths?"

"I'm sure they would," Gabe said.

She nodded. "And the drug company has been putting pressure on you to keep quiet?"

"They have indeed." He explained about the censorship at the *Chronicle,* the canceled TV news story, and the drugs planted in his hospital locker.

"These corporate execs don't like whistle-blowers" she said. She caught the waiter's eye across the room and made a gesture of writing on her upraised hand. "But we do. We like to protect them and help them get their say. This dry-cleaning lady in San Diego," she said. "What's her name?"

"Hattie Mae Davis."

"You think she'd go on camera and tell us about her experience?"

Gabe nodded. "I think she would. I'd be glad to ask."

"A first-person description of what the headache feels like to the victim would be great television."

"She's good," Gabe said. "You'll like her. I'll give

you a call after I talk to her. You want to give me a number where I can reach you?"

Monica shook her head. "I'll call you," she said. "I'm going to be on the road the rest of the week." She took a long swallow of coffee. "You may be right." She smiled, an impish look coming onto her face. "I'm beginning to think this *is* our kind of story."

A steady rain fell as Gabe drove back to his apartment. He was surprised to find Kate's Saab in the parking space in front of his uncle's store. The shock of seeing her here made his insides spasm. *Don't go jumping to conclusions,* he told himself. *Remember— she works for Kimberley now*. He put his car in the garage and came in quietly through the back, pausing at the storeroom door.

Kate was behind the pharmacy counter, in animated conversation with his uncle. He could not make out what they were saying. He glanced past them into the front of the store. A heavyset teenager in a Lincoln High athletic jacket lurked near the condoms. A pale blond woman in a long green coat was comparing two bottles of baby shampoo.

His uncle saw him first. He put a hand on Kate's shoulder and turned her toward the rear door.

When Kate saw him her mouth dropped open and her lower lip began to tremble. "Gabe?"

"Hi, baby. I've been trying to reach you."

"I . . . I know," she said. "I'm sorry. I kind of freaked out there for a while."

She moved toward him. He opened his arms to her. Gabe closed his eyes and held on tight. It felt like home.

"Oh, babes. I really blew it, didn't I?" She nuzzled at his shoulder. Gabe's uncle was wiping his glasses with a handkerchief, his eyes glistening with unaccustomed emotion.

"They've really gone crazy out there," she said. "I never would have thought—"

"Why? What's happened?" Gabe said, aware of the suspicion in his voice. "Why the sudden change?"

She looked up at him, her face soft and vulnerable. "I guess I deserve that. I was pretty stupid . . ." She took Gabe's hands and pressed them to her lips.

"They *have* been receiving adverse-drug-reaction reports," she said. "Ed has been hiding them. And he staged that phony press conference just to find out how much you knew and to get the footage of all his top executives taking Virazine."

"Did you really take active Virazine?" Gabe asked her. "Are you feeling okay?"

"I'm fine, but somebody at the company sent me copies of three hidden ADRs. I've got them with me. Howard went nuts when I told him. He kept saying this was exactly what he'd warned them about. He confronted Ed about it. He said he was going to call you and offer you the story. Did he ever . . ."

Gabe shook his head. "I haven't heard from him."

"I haven't either," Kate said. "It's so odd. He's disappeared. I can't find him anywhere."

"You mean he's out of his laminar-flow room?"

She nodded. "Yes, he's gone. He's off his medication, so he could be anywhere. He usually touches base with me at least once a day when he's away from the lab, but I haven't heard from him since the day before yesterday. There was no answer at your place so I called your uncle. He told me your apartment had been broken into. I was afraid they might have taken you, too."

"My apartment?" he said.

It appeared as if someone had taken a baseball bat to the place. The front door of Gabe's apartment hung diagonally from its upper hinge. His computer lay on its side on the floor, a dark jagged hole where the screen had been. Silver shards of glass covered the room like a light snowfall. The drawers of his filing cabinets had been overturned on the floor. His books had been swept off the shelves, the drawers of his desk kicked to splinters among the rubble.

His answering machine had been knocked to the floor, but it was still plugged in and the message light was on. Gabe pressed the Play button.

"Hey, Gabe, baby. Marty Dorland at the *Chron*. We've been getting a lot of pressure from our legal department. I'm afraid the features editor has decided to put your column on hold until all this blows over. I trust it'll all be okay. Talk with you soon."

"Terrific," Gabe said. "Three out of three. Suspended from the hospital, off the station, and out of a newspaper column. They're really hitting all the bases."

Kate frowned. "You've been suspended from the hospital?"

Gabe nodded. "They planted some stolen drugs in my locker."

"And how about this?" She gestured across the debris of the ruined office. "I mean, I guess Ed probably ordered it, but who actually did it?"

"Two candidates I can think of. I'm pretty sure Chip Downey was in here once before. And Sheila said she heard Ed talking about this hit man named Santini."

Kate's face darkened. "Sheila's on their side," Kate said. "She's a very crazy woman, Gabe. I think she's involved in this. Who's this Santini supposed to be?"

"Some thug, I think. I gather they've asked him to try to scare me off the case. That's not all they're doing, either." He described his meeting with Ray Brody. "He said there'd be some real heat if I didn't behave myself. I guess this is what he meant."

Kate shook her head. "I never thought Ed would do anything like this." She let out a long breath, shaking her head sadly. "Do you want to look at the ADRs?"

"Sure."

"There was a note with them. Here." She handed him a piece of yellow paper.

Dear Dr. Reiley,
I came across the originals of these by accident and I'm so upset I don't know what to do. They were in the bottom drawer of Dr. McCauley's private filing cabinet. I'm enclosing an extra copy of the key. Sorry to drop this in your lap like this, but I have kids to support and I'm afraid for my job. I'm hoping and praying you'll do the right thing. Sorry I can't sign my name to this.

—A friend

Gabe glanced quickly through the reports. They were from Pittsburgh, New Orleans, and Seattle. All three patients had died of complications of high blood pressure. All had been taking Virazine.

"I'm sending copies to the FDA and *60 Minutes* right now," he said. "They're not going to be able to sit on this any longer."

"*60 Minutes?*"

Gabe nodded. "I'll tell you about it on the way to Howard's place."

The midday traffic was light across the Golden Gate Bridge. As they reached the north tower, Kate pulled her Saab into the right-hand lane.

"The finish line for the marathon will be right over there," she said. She pointed over at the view spot on the Sausalito side of the bridge. "You still up for riding with me?"

"Wouldn't miss it," Gabe said.

"So tell me about the woman from *60 Minutes.*"

He told her all the way north on 101 and onto the Tiburon exit. Tiburon Boulevard ran east of the freeway, out to the northern coast of San Francisco Bay. They followed the bay road north.

"60 Minutes. That would be something," Kate said. "Think they're really going to do it?"

Gabe shrugged. "Monica Penny seemed pretty enthusiastic. It would sure help if Howard would go on camera."

"I'll bet he will, if we can find him," Kate said. "Howard is one of the most fearless people I've ever known. Here we are."

She pulled up beside an old duplex covered with gray shingles and supported by thick black pilings. A large, weathered deck on each unit extended out over a rocky little beach that edged San Pablo Bay. Far out across the water they could make out the dark shape of the East Bay.

"Nice view," Gabe said.

"Yeah," Kate said. "It looks great, but it's actually cold and damp as hell. Wait a minute." She opened the trunk, took out a black canvas jacket, and put it on. Gabe stopped and put his arms around her.

"What is it?" she said.

"Guilt. I've been entertaining a bad fantasy."

"What?" Her eyes searched his, suddenly afraid.

"I shouldn't tell you," he said.

"Please."

He let out a long breath. "I was thinking that maybe you were going to take me up some dark alley where this Santini would beat the shit out of me."

"Oh, Gabe." She put her arms around him, her temple under his jaw. "I'm sorry. I really let you down, didn't I?"

Gabe smiled, stroking her hair. "It's great to have you back on my side. I was thinking of giving the whole thing up."

"No! You can't." Her eyes were wide with indignation. "I won't let you. Too many people have died, Gabe. You've got to stay with this."

He wrapped his arms around her waist and planted a kiss on her neck. "Okay," he said. "I will."

A wooden wheelchair ramp—a recent addition— led down the left side of the building to the front deck of the lower unit. The old porch sagged under their weight. There were no lights on in the house. No one answered their knock.

"He may still be asleep," Kate said. "He works all night sometimes." She knocked again.

Gabe peered into a dark window at his reflection. "Have you been in here before?"

She nodded. "I've driven him home a couple of times."

"I think we should go in and take a look," Gabe said.

"That won't be so easy. Howard's pretty security conscious."

"Imagine that you're Howard," Gabe said "Where would you hide an extra key?"

"Somewhere you could get to from a wheelchair."

"Take a look. I'll check out the front door."

He heard her walking slowly up the steps. The door had a cylinder lock surrounded by a brass armored plate. The frame was solid metal, the strikeplate of the lock protected by a thick flange of stainless steel.

"No key I can find," Kate said, coming back to the porch. "The people upstairs aren't home. Here's the tool kit from my car."

"We'd need a locksmith or a cutting torch to get in this way," Gabe said. "Let's see what else we've got."

It took Gabe fifteen minutes to scout out all the windows and doors around the building. He finally settled on a bathroom window he could reach from the deck.

He rolled a wire-spool table beneath the window, got out his pocket knife, and began chipping the brittle, salt-hardened putty away from the yellowed glass. It took him nearly half an hour to pry the pane lose. He slipped the glass free and handed it down to Kate.

"Success," she said.

"We're not in yet."

She took the sharp rectangle of glass and placed it carefully on the deck. "I was afraid a cop was going to drive by."

Gabe reached in through the open pane and found the window lock. "Oh, great. It's the kind that locks with a key. I'm getting tired of this. You want to give me that big screwdriver?"

She handed it up to him. "What are you going to do?"

"Bust this sucker off." He positioned the screwdriver blade between the lock and the window sash and twisted. He heard the wood splinter. The lock fell to the floor inside. Gabe pried up the lower sash and put his head into the open window. "I'll meet you at the front door," he said.

The apartment smelled damp and musty. Gabe stepped down on the washbasin and made a quick survey of the place. It was a messy, rambling two-bedroom unit. Half the furniture appeared to have come from Goodwill, the other half from Neiman-Marcus. He made his way to the front door.

There was a key on the inside of the lock. He opened the door and Kate stepped in and made a face.

"Jesus," she said. "It smells like a clam's laundry in here."

"Looks like he's had the same visitors I did," Gabe said.

"Oh, no." Kate followed him to the back bedroom. A large computer workstation dominated the room. Three floppy-disk cases stood on the table beside it, their lids tipped back like the dislocated jaws of so many dark, square skulls. They were all empty. The drawers of the desk had been ransacked. Papers covered the floor.

Kate frowned and disappeared into the bathroom. She came back a moment later, saying, "He took his syringes and insulin with him."

Gabe nodded. "That's a good sign. Let's take a look at the computer." Gabe sat down at the desk chair. The disk drive was empty; the directory of the hard disk was blank.

"Looks like they've erased everything," Gabe said.

"Isn't that a little delicate for thugs? Why didn't they just take it?"

"Probably trying to make it look like a routine robbery," Gabe replied. "Your ordinary burglar wouldn't know where to unload a specialized piece of gear like this."

"So the files are gone for good?" Kate said.

"Maybe not. When you erase a hard disk it doesn't actually destroy the files. It just erases the directory and eventually the old files get written over by new ones. Let me pop out the hard disk and see if Lu Jean can figure out how to get them back."

Two hours later Gabe was sitting on a hard wooden chair at the Lincoln High School computer lab looking out the window. He saw Kate moving steadily around the track outside. The fan in Lu Jean's workstation hummed in harmony with the drone of the fluorescent lights.

"How much longer do you think it's going to be?" he asked.

Lu Jean looked up from the computer keyboard and smiled, the bright hues of the color monitor reflecting off her glasses. "Stop fidgeting, boss. I think I have the whole directory now."

"You sure?"

Lu Jean nodded. "It's only a thousand meg drive and I've got nine hundred twenty megs already."

"Let's take a look," Gabe said.

"They look like the names of drugs or chemicals or something," Lu Jean said.

Gabe scanned the file list for Virazine or riboxyuridine. He opened files with names he didn't recognize. The last listing on the directory was a file named Zap. When she attempted to open the file, she got a dialogue box requesting a password.

"Not good," Gabe said. "Doesn't look like we're going to be able to get in."

"Hold on. Let me look at the code." Lu Jean opened another file and hit a sequence of keys. This brought up a long list of programming commands. She scrolled quickly through the list.

"It's written in C," she said. "There's a lot of complicated graphics stuff in there. Oh, yeah. I see what he did. Look. See there? The password is 'whistle.' "

"How do you know that?"

"It's right there in the program code."

A program-loading message remained on the screen for some time. When the screen finally cleared, the machine began running a three-dimensional sequence, complete with a computer-generated voice:

This is the molecule 7-(3-nitrophenyl)-riboxyhy-

drazide, known generically as riboxyuridine. This molecule is now trademarked under the name Virazine.

"Bingo," Gabe said.

An image of the molecule appeared, a long, green complex like some thick, branching undersea plant. It slowly began to rotate.

"Damn. You got it. Great work, kiddo." Gabe pulled up his chair beside Lu Jean's, watching in fascination as the ghostly molecule moved across the screen.

As I noted in my initial report, this molecule bears a striking similarity to another molecule, trans-2-methyl-3-nitrocarboxylic acid 3-riboxybenzylhydrazide, a powerful monoamine oxidase inhibitor. The screen went blank. Then another, similar molecule appeared, this one in light blue. Where the long end of the first molecule was bulb-shaped, the right end of the second was shaped like a Y. It too began to rotate.

The bioconversion from the cis form to the trans configuration is actively promoted in the presence of high concentrations of the enzyme xanthosine reductase.

The first molecule reappeared. A small round red glob—evidently representing the enzyme—drifted in over the molecule's green body and covered the bulb-shaped end. There was a flash on the screen and a sound like a cork coming out of a bottle. The enzyme drifted away. They saw that the molecule had been converted into the forked, blue form.

We looked very closely for such a reaction during the preclinical phase and . . . The sound track stopped abruptly. The screen went blank except for a blinking cursor and the message:

SYNTAX ERROR IN LINE 10220

Gabe put a hand on Lu Jean's shoulder. "That's all?"

"Let's look at that line." Lu Jean typed in a command. The screen cleared, then flashed:

```
10220 GOSUB 20500
```

Lu Jean opened the program code and scrolled far down into the program.

"There's no subroutine 20500 to go to," she said at last. "Either he was still working on it, or this was just an early draft."

35

Gabe was afraid they would be stopped at the door. But the Kimberley guard, a silent, thick-fingered man with a bad complexion, pushed a visitor's badge across the desk and waved them through.

Kate leaned back against the wall of the elevator and let out a long breath. "I sure hope he's down there," she said.

"I can't believe they'd do anything to Howard," Gabe said. "Talk about killing the goose that lays the golden eggs."

The hallway smelled of ozone and alcohol. Howard's door was unlocked. Inside, they heard a deep rumbling.

"That's a good sign," Kate said. "Maybe he had a flare-up and had to get back in a hurry."

They put on masks and gloves and went in. The wall of plastic strips rose to greet them. Gabe felt the warm wind on his face.

Howard's office appeared much the same as it had on their previous visit. The lights were low, the computer screens dark.

"Not here," Kate said, lowering her voice. "Maybe he's in back."

He followed her to the door in the back wall. She knocked, waited for an answer, then opened it. They looked in at a modest bedroom with a dresser and a single bed. There was another door in the back of the room.

"The bathroom?" Gabe asked.

Kate nodded.

The bathroom door was not quite closed. Gabe pushed it open. It was dark and humid inside, full of a strange, sweet smell. Gabe felt the hair standing up on the back of his neck. He flipped the light switch, but the room remained in darkness.

"There's a funny smell in here." he said. He was finding it difficult to breathe.

"What's the matter?"

"I don't know. The light's out. Have you got your penlight?"

She dug in her purse and handed it to him. He pointed it into the darkness. The shower curtain had been pulled across the tub. It bore bright images of Donald Duck with his nephews, Huey, Louie, and Dewey, Daisy Duck, Uncle Scrooge, and Gladstone Gander, all printed in bright primary colors. Gabe's foot slipped on the wet tile. He took a deep breath and pulled back the curtain.

Howard lay absolutely still, his eyes wide open, staring dreamily up at the ceiling from beneath the gray film of the bath water. He was floating on his back, his one leg bent beneath him at a sharp angle, so that his left kneecap touched the drain under the spigot. His long hair spread out in the water above his head. His body was white and still in the glare of the penlight.

"Oh, Jesus," Gabe said. He raised his arm, trying to shield Kate from the sight, but she had pushed in beside him.

"Oh my God," Kate said. "Oh my good God." They both stared down at the motionless figure.

It seemed to Gabe as if they had stepped into a kind of three-dimensional tableau, the air frozen around them like one of those childhood Christmas scenes locked inside a glass ball. Kate made a retching sound and stumbled from the room. He could hear her sobbing and vomiting outside.

Gabe forced himself to look down at the corpse in the bathtub. Howard lay pale, peaceful, and unmoving in the still water, his long face thoughtful, his eyes wide with wonder, as if he had been overtaken at the moment of death by some wild joy. *Easy,* he told himself. *Easy now. Pay attention.*

He looked away from the dead man, forcing himself to examine the room. A syringe and two clear glass vials lay on the tile counter beside a red toothbrush and a large tube of Crest. A white comb that needed cleaning lay beside a bundle of Q-Tips held by a rubber band. He looked back at the tub, mentally blocking out the image of the body in order to focus on its surroundings. It was only then that he saw that there was a small radio in the bottom of the tub, its cord still plugged into an electric socket above the counter.

He found Kate leaning on the wall, sobbing, her hands over her face. She shook her head and slipped her arms around his waist. Gabe looked across her shoulder into the eyes of another poster of Einstein, riding a bicycle. Above his head was a hand-lettered dialogue balloon: *Science should be explained in terms as simple as possible. But no simpler.*

He held her. After a few moments she drew a deep breath.

"You okay?" he said.

She nodded. "Do . . . do you think . . ."

Gabe had passed through the first shock and could feel the anger rising inside him. "Look around and see if anything's missing, but don't touch anything," he said. "I'm going to call Pat Ditmore at the sheriff's office."

Gabe had just finished dialing when the door burst open. Chip Downey stood in the doorway, holding a black automatic in a two-handed marksman's stance. The gun looked like a toy in his massive hands. Two dark-uniformed figures hovered behind him.

"Hold it," he ordered them. "Security."

"Oh, Mr. Downey. Thank God you're here," Kate said, ignoring the gun. She held back the plastic strips to let him in. "There's been an awful accident. Howard Pearlman is dead."

Downey lowered his gun. "Pearlman? Dead? Jesus." He appeared genuinely stunned. "What the hell's happening down here, Doctor?" he asked. "I got a report of an unauthorized . . ."

"That's him right there, chief." The security guard who had been at the desk stepped forward, pointing at Gabe. "There was a picture of him up on our bulletin board. I had to go back and look again—"

"Shut up, Stewart. I know who he is," Downey said. He put the gun into his shoulder holster and rubbed his hand absently across his bald spot. "What's this about Pearlman?"

"Back here," Gabe said. "We just found him."

"Where?" Downey came toward him, patting the bulge under his arm.

Gabe tapped at the phone receiver. "I'm talking to Lieutenant Ditmore at the sheriff's office," he said. He spoke into the phone. "Pat? It's Chip Downey, Kimberley's head of security. He just busted in. Yeah, sure. Hold on."

Gabe held out the phone to Downey. "He wants to talk to you."

Downey took the receiver, listened, and made compliant noises. He nodded several times and hung up, raising his thick eyebrows.

"Lieutenant Ditmore wants me to keep everybody on ice until his people get here," he said. "Stewart and Pomeroy. Outside. Nobody in or out until the deputies get here. One of you doctors want to show me the deceased?"

Ditmore arrived twenty minutes later. He was a deliberate man of forty-five with a tan, weathered face. He wore cowboy boots and a western-cut suit that was tight in the shoulders. His hat had left a shiny crease in his thinning gray-brown hair. He looked from Gabe to Kate with his mild blue eyes.

"Gabe. How are you?" he said. "And this must be Dr. Reiley." He moved to shake hands, then stopped suddenly. "What's with the gloves?" he asked. Kate explained.

"AIDS, huh? I guess you might as well get me

some gloves too:" Ditmore cleared his throat and introduced his two assistants. The first was a tall, red-haired young woman with a camera; the second, a scrawny young man wearing glasses and holding a heavy aluminum case.

"Let me take a quick look, then you guys can go ahead and get to work," Ditmore said. The technician held open a pair of rubber gloves and Ditmore slipped his hands into them and pulled them tight.

"You'll need a light," Gabe said. "There's a blown fuse in there."

Ditmore got a black flashlight from the evidence box and went into the bathroom. Gabe squeezed in beside him.

"Anybody touch anything?"

"Just the shower curtain," Gabe said.

Ditmore pointed the flashlight beam down at the radio under the bath water. "What do you think, it fell in on top of him?"

"I think somebody threw it in later, to make it look like an accident."

Ditmore pointed at the two glass vials on the counter. "What's in those?"

"Insulin," Gabe said. "He was a diabetic."

"A diabetic AIDS patient, huh?"

Gabe nodded. "Injected himself several times a day, or had somebody else . . ."

"Hello, you two. What have we got here?" Loren Price, the county coroner, stood in the doorway. He was short and florid and stout in a crisp gray flannel suit that hung a little loosely. He carried two large black leather bags.

"Hello, Doc," Ditmore said. "You know Dr. Gabe Austin and Dr. Kate Reiley, here?"

"By reputation. Glad to meet you both." His hand

was soft and chilly. He was breathing hard. There was a liquid tremor in his eye.

Ditmore gave him a look of genuine concern. "You okay, Doc? I hear you've been pretty busy."

Price nodded ruefully. "Big bus accident up by Ignacio," he said. "Sixteen schoolchildren hurt and three killed. A hell of a mess. What have you got for me here?"

"A dead man in a bathtub," Ditmore said. "An AIDS patient no less. Got an electric radio hanging in the tub with him."

The breaker had been reset and the light was working. The crime-lab people had taken the radio, the vials, the syringe, and the toilet articles. Only the body was left. Price had taken a Polaroid camera out of his bag and was shooting flash pictures of the body.

"The lieutenant said you wanted to sit in with me while I examine the body," Price said. He knelt on the bathroom floor, opening his bag.

"If you don't mind," Gabe said. He took a deep breath, letting it out slowly through pursed lips. Kate had said that she would wait for him in her office.

"Glad to have the company. You can help me lift him. Better put on a second pair of gloves." Gabe shook out another pair of gloves and slipped them on.

Price took out a second Poloroid camera and began taking pictures of the scene. "These are just for my own records," he said. "I have a very visual mind. One look at one of my files and I can go back and remember a whole case."

"You must have quite a collection," Gabe said.

"Oh, yes. I get them all," Price said. "The auto

accidents. The domestic killings. The drug shoot-outs. The bridge jumpers that wash up on the north shore. We get two or three bathtub drownings a year. Usually involve alcohol. Mmmm. The water's down to room temperature. He's been in there five or six hours at least."

He recorded his finding in a black notebook, took off his jacket, rolled up his sleeves, dipped a sample of the bath water into a glass vial, and pushed the lever that opened the drain. They watched as the body—it seemed clear to Gabe that it was no longer a person now—settled slowly to the bottom of the tub.

The body was surprisingly heavy and stiff. It was like lifting a cement statue. With some difficulty they hoisted the corpse over the side of the tub and lowered it to the bathroom floor.

"Body temperature first," Price said. He picked up a body temperature punch, a long chrome instrument that looked like a fat ice pick. Gabe looked away. There was a sound like a knife going into a ripe melon as Price drove the punch into the upper right abdomen. When he looked back, Price was inserting a long industrial thermometer.

"Room temperature," he said at last. "Make that nine or ten hours."

36

The yellow note taped to the office door directed Gabe and Kate back to Gertrude's private lab. They found her working at the negative-pressure hood, a small, enclosed, glass-walled room built around a high lab bench. Gertrude's work sometimes required the use of nerve gas, powerful acids, and other hazardous substances. A powerful exhaust fan inside the sealed, glass-walled room sucked away the toxic fumes.

"She looks so content," Gabe whispered. "I hate to interrupt her." He reached out and tapped gently on the glass.

Gertrude raised a hand in greeting, capped a big bottle of acid, and came out to them.

"Ah. There you are," she said, raising her voice to be heard over the low hiss of the negative-pressure system. She wore a long white lab coat over a bright flowered dress. "And you brought your friend Kate. How wonderful."

She closed the heavy glass door behind her, picked up her cane, and shuffled across to shake Kate's hand.

"Hello, Gertrude," Kate said. "It's been a long time."

"Yes, yes. Too many years. And how healthy you look." Gertrude nodded approvingly. "I can see you are living a life that is very good for you. And you have become a famous runner now. We are all so . . ." She stopped, looking quickly back and forth between them. "But what is it? What's wrong?"

"Gertrude." He put his hand on her arm. "Howard Pearlman is dead."

"Oh no." The expression on Gertrude's face changed from affection to dismay. "That sweet boy. Was it . . ."

Gabe shook his head. "We think he was murdered," he said.

"Murdered?" Gertrude blinked as if she had been exposed to a bright light.

Gabe nodded. "He'd threatened to blow the whistle on the company. He'd even written a computer program describing an alternate pathway that would convert Virazine into an MAO inhibitor."

"But who would do such a thing?" Gertrude shook her head.

Kate took her arm. "Gertrude, I hate to say it, but Ed Elias is acting like a total corporate scumbag." She and Gabe brought Gertrude up to date on the break-ins, the threats, the planted drugs, and the censorship at the TV station and the newspaper.

"They've got Ray Brody pulling every string he can to cover this whole thing up," Gabe said. "And we've had warnings that they've brought in an outside muscle guy to shut me up for good."

Gertrude's eyes brightened when Gabe described his visit with Monica Penny. "But this is good," she said. "You say that Howard spoke of an alternative breakdown pattern. We must find the mechanism."

Gabe nodded. "It's our best chance. If we can show how it works on *60 Minutes,* it'll be all over.

The drug will be off the market within a couple of days.''

"All right," Gertrude said. "Let's get to work. Were you able to establish an MAO trigger substance for each of your cases?"

Gabe nodded. "Every one I've looked into so far."

"Good. I think we're really closing in," Gertrude said. "Did you remember to stop at the deli?"

"Got it right here." Gabe placed the white-wrapped package on the black, waist-high lab bench. "What have you done so far?"

Gertrude settled herself on a high metal stool. "I've analyzed all the samples for contamination. We found nothing. I think we can cross that off our list."

"Okay," Gabe said. "That's some progress."

Gertrude led them to a set of cages on a low cart. "Two days ago, Gabe and I inoculated these mousies with a new herpes culture they just isolated at the University of Washington," she said. "One day ago, no more food. Water only, poor things. Now we give them little rat-doses of this pill you are suspecting."

"So you're testing to see whether this new herpes strain could be the missing link?" Kate asked.

Gabe nodded. He felt happy to be in the safe, secure laboratory. He wanted to stay there, doing the experiments that would bring the whole thing to a conclusion.

"Gertrude, I think we need to do something more." Gabe said. "I've been thinking about this for the last few days, ever since I was helping you . . ."

"Yes." Gertrude smiled. "I know what you are thinking."

"You do?"

She nodded. "I saw how you 'accidentally' inoculated yourself with the new herpes culture."

"So what do you think?" Gabe asked, looking

back and forth between Kate and Gertrude. "After all, rats aren't people."

"Gabe?" Kate shook her head. "What are you talking about?"

"He is talking about running this experiment on himself," Gertrude said.

"I've brought along everything we'd need." Gabe opened his briefcase, taking out a selection of syringes, a blood pressure cuff, and a white deli bag.

Kate's mouth gaped open. "Gabe, please don't joke," she said.

"I'm perfectly serious," he said. "I've got a good supply of Regitine right here. And I've got both of you standing by to reverse the MAO reaction if it does occur. After all, you've taken Virazine yourself."

"But deliberately trying to provoke a reaction?" Kate shook her head. "Gertrude, don't let him do it."

Gabe turned to the old woman. "What do you think?"

Gertrude leaned forward on her cane. "We could reverse an MAO inhibitor reaction, I suppose." Her grin broke through her reserve. "It would be just like the old days," she said. "Back when I was in school in Germany, my professors and I used to try these drugs ourselves all the time."

Gertrude had the Virazine solution already made up. Gabe would hand her a rat, she would pry open its mouth, slip the eyedropper between its lips, and squeeze the drug into its mouth, then hold its mouth closed and stroke it under the chin until it had swallowed every drop. Kate took the rats and placed them in a large common cage. They repeated the procedure for each of the dozen rats.

Gabe unwrapped the two-pound chunk of aged

cheddar. He opened the door, shooed the rats away from the opening, and pushed the wedge of cheese into the center of the cage. The rats sniffed the cheese cautiously at first, as if they could not believe their good fortune. A small black-and-white male took a tentative bite. Eventually they all set to work in earnest. The mountain of cheese began to shrink before their eyes.

"My turn now," Gabe said. Gertrude had measured out a small beaker of cloudy fluid.

"Here is your cocktail," she said.

"Gabe. You're sure?" Kate put out a hand to touch his cheek.

He took her hand. "It's a small enough risk. And if it can really make the difference . . ." He searched her face. "But I won't do it unless it's okay with you."

She shook her head. "Do what you think is best," she said. "I'm just scared for you, that's all."

"Yeah. Me too." He lifted the glass vessel in his hand. It had a slight salty-lemon smell. "Why the liquid?" Gabe said. "What's wrong with the pills?"

"This is quicker," Gertrude said. "We don't have to wait for the pills to dissolve."

Kate took his hand.

"All right then. Down the hatch." He brought the beaker to his lips and drank the liquid. It was room temperature and tasted like an old-fashioned lemon-quinine concoction.

Gertrude took the vial from his hands. She carried it to the sink and rinsed it out. "And what will you take for your high-tyramine food?"

Gabe licked his lips. His head was beginning to ache ever so slightly. He told himself it had to be his imagination. He hadn't even eaten the trigger food yet.

"Got it right here," he said, with a good deal more enthusiasm than he felt. From the white deli sack he removed a six-ounce bottle of pickled herring.

"That should do it, don't you think?"

"Oh, yes," Gertrude said. "Pickled herring has more tyramine than practically anything."

"Gabe?" Kate was looking across at him, tears in her eyes. "We could still just walk away from all this. Are you sure?"

Gabe shook his head. "It's way past that, I'm afraid." He uncapped the bottle, got out the plastic fork, and began eating his way through the jar of herring.

"Now what?" Kate asked, glancing back at Gertrude.

Gertrude smiled. "Now you take his blood pressure. And we wait."

The readings started out nearly normal, but after twenty minutes Gabe could tell from the look on Kate's face that they had begun to go up. After the tenth reading, she handed the pad to Gertrude. Gabe craned his neck to get a glimpse. The latest reading was 155/110. Definitely much too high.

Gertrude put a calming hand on Gabe's shoulder and peered down at the blood pressure chart.

"Excuse me, Gabe, but, Kate, you must not let him see what readings you are getting anymore," Gertrude said.

"What do you mean?" Kate said. "Why not?"

Gertrude shook her head. "We must do everything we can to avoid a white-coat reaction." In a white-coat reaction, anxiety increases blood pressure.

Gertrude put her hands on Gabe's neck, massaging his tense muscles. He realized that she was attempting to calm him with her touch, as she quieted her lab animals.

"Gabe, you must sit very quietly and relax as much as you can. Close your eyes. Take deep breaths. Pretend that you are visiting a favorite spot. A place you feel perfectly safe and secure. A place where you can completely relax. And visualize your blood pressure being nice and low."

Gertrude remained behind him, her hands on his shoulders. Gabe closed his eyes and went into a dark, quiet inner space. He stayed that way for a long time, Gertrude's hands on his shoulders, Kate working the blood pressure cuff on his arm.

After what seemed a very long time, Gertrude said, "You know, I think we are all right now."

"Yes," Kate said. "It looks okay, doesn't it?"

"Can I look?" Gabe asked.

"Yes. You are back to normal," Gertrude said.

Gabe looked across at the blood pressure record. It started out at 118 over 86, went up as high as 160 over 118, then gradually returned to 122 over 88.

Gabe turned to Gertrude. "That look like an anxiety reaction to you?"

She nodded. "Yes. And understandably so. As soon as you began to relax, it started coming down."

"How about the rats?" Gabe asked.

Gertrude laughed. "Yes, we forgot all about the poor mousies."

They hurried to the cage. The rats had long since devoured the cheese and had gone off to the various corners of the cage to nap and to lick themselves.

They waited late into the night, rechecking Gabe's blood pressure, drinking tea, and watching the rats closely for any sign of difficulty. But both the rats and Gabe remained perfectly happy and content. It was well after midnight when they finally declared the experiment a failure.

Driving back to Fairfax—Kate was already asleep in the seat beside him—Gabe didn't know whether to feel relieved or disappointed. He felt both happy and sad—disappointed that they had not yet reached a solution, happy that he and Gertrude and Kate were working together. He could only hope that with a little more time they would find the answer.

The ringing phone jarred Gabe awake. He groped for the receiver in the darkness. Gertrude's excited voice brought him to immediate attention.

"Gabe, I think perhaps I have the answer. Can you come over right away?"

"You're still at the lab?"

"Yes."

"What time is it?"

"Just after five-thirty. I am sorry to call so early . . ."

"Kate just went out to run. Give us an hour and a half."

"Hurry," she said. "It's too exciting to keep."

It was 6:55 A.M. when they pulled into the Parnassus Street parking garage. The pharmacology lab was completely quiet, the centrifuges still, the computers dark. The same note was still taped to the office door. But the door to Gertrude's private lab was locked.

"That's odd," Gabe said.

"Maybe she just ran out for a minute," Kate said.

Gabe shook his head. "That doesn't make sense. She said she was going to wait for us. Let me try my key." The key turned easily in the lock. As he started to turn the knob he was aware of an old familiar odor. He jerked the door shut.

"Nerve gas. Back. Back!" He grabbed Kate around the waist and pulled her away from the door. "We've got to get out of here. Fast. Are you okay?"

"I'm fine." She looked at him closely, her eyes widening with sudden concern. "Gabe. What's the matter? You look awful."

"I got a whiff of it," he said. He felt his chest tightening. His nose was running. His vision was beginning to blur.

"Gabe! Are you . . ."

"I can't see. You're going to have to help me. Hit the fire alarm. Then get me to the elevator." His voice sounded remarkably calm.

Gabe heard Kate's rapid breathing in the darkness. There was the sound of the glass of the fire alarm breaking. Kate took his arm and led him down the hall.

"How about Gertrude?" she said.

"If she's in there it's already too late."

As the elevator descended he heard the fire bells going off on the other floors.

It seemed to Gabe that all the fluids were desperately trying to make their way out of his body. Kate had to lead him across the street to the men's room in the student union. He locked himself in a stall. It was a good twenty minutes before the worst of it was over, the tears and the salivation, the runny nose and the diarrhea. As he waited, his vision gradually returned.

By the time he was able to make his way back out to the street, two police cruisers had closed down Parnassus Street from Third to Arguello. Uniformed patrolmen were putting up a line of white police barriers.

Kate was talking with a short, friendly man with a walrus mustache. She greeted Gabe with a hug.

"You okay?" she said.

"Yeah. We were lucky. One more step. That would have been it." He blew his nose on a paper towel.

"Dr. Austin? I'm Jesse Hernandez. Homicide division. Captain Perkins asked me to come check this out. You need some medical attention?"

"I'll be okay," Gabe said. "But I'm worried about Gertrude. I'm pretty sure she's still inside. Have you got some way to blow that stuff out of there?"

Hernandez shook his head. "My orders are to secure the building. Nobody goes in until the poison control people get here."

"But there's someone in there," Kate said. "There must be something . . ."

"Sorry, ma'm. Orders are orders." Hernandez turned to Gabe. "What makes you think it was a homicide?"

Gabe looked up at the building and shook his head. "Gertrude was too smart to make a mistake with nerve gas. Besides, she was investigating something really hot. She called us at five-thirty this morning to say that she'd had some kind of breakthrough. The matter she was looking into could have cost a certain drug company several hundred million dollars."

Hernandez looked thoughtful. "What is nerve gas, anyway? Some kind of poison?"

Gabe nodded. "It's one of the most toxic substances known to science."

"What are the symptoms?" Hernandez looked at him closely, as if trying to evaluate whether the drug might have affected his mind.

"In a small dose, like I got, runny nose, tearing, sweating, salivation, intestinal cramps, and big-time diarrhea."

"And a big dose?"

Gabe shook his head, remembering a film he had seen the previous year. Saddam Hussein had used nerve gas to execute a group of condemned prisoners and had filmed the result. It had not been a pleasant thing to watch.

"You get an almost instantaneous discharge of all bodily fluids," he said. "Vomiting. Tearing. Salivation. Diarrhea. Uncontrollable urination. You froth at the mouth and go into convulsions. Then you stop breathing."

"Jesus." Hernandez took an involuntary step away from the building.

A big white van from the San Francisco Poison Control Center pulled up beside them. Jules Wolfe got out, followed by two young technicians. Jules was a thin, youthful man of forty with light mahogany skin and a natural, fluid grace. He was the best industrial toxicologist in the state.

"Hey there, Gabe." Wolfe gestured up at the windows of the pharmacology lab. "You really got a nerve gas leak up there?"

"Yeah. And Gertrude Potter is still up there, Julie. We've got to get her out."

Wolfe raised his eyebrows. "Not someone you'd think would make a mistake with nerve gas. All right.

We'll get out the robot. And you'll all have to put these on." He handed them each a gas mask.

Hernandez dangled his mask from a strap, eyeing it suspiciously. "You serious, Doc? We really have to do this?"

Wolfe looked at him sharply. "Either that or get out of the area. You don't mess around with this stuff," Wolfe said. He made a waving motion to the technicians in the truck. "You know what kind it is?"

"VX," Gabe said. "Commercial grade."

Wolfe nodded grimly. "You're lucky. You got a little warning. If it was GB you'd both be dead."

"Can you test for VX?" Gabe said.

Wolfe shrugged. "It says in the book we can. It's actually a test for something else, but the organophosphates are supposed to bump it up a little. I guess we'll see."

Hernandez tugged at his mask. "Suppose your test doesn't pick it up. How do we know when it's safe?"

Wolfe smiled. He gestured back over his shoulder toward the two technicians. "That's what I bring these guys for."

Gabe went across the street and attempted to call Gertrude's lab and office. There was no answer. When he got back, Wolfe and his asistants were still working to get the machine ready. Gabe paced back and forth beside the truck, sweaty and soiled.

At last the two technicians, masked and suited, rolled the heavy stainless-steel device out onto the tailgate, then lowered it slowly to the ground. It looked like a miniature tank with a video camera on top and folded metal arms at the sides.

One of the techs used the on-board control panel to maneuver the cart to the front door. Then he and his partner went back to the van and wheeled out another cart full of equipment, this one tethered to the van by a long bundle of black wires.

"Okay, Lieutenant," Wolfe said. "If you'd be good enough to open that door for us, we'll see if we can figure out what's happening in there."

Hernandez held open the door. Wolfe punched a sequence of keys and pushed the joystick forward. The motor began to whir and the treads began to turn. The cart moved slowly into the lobby.

"Over here," Wolfe said. "We can watch it on the monitor."

Two floodlights on the cart came on, lighting up the lobby. The camera panned the room slowly, showing them the building directory, then a wall full of posters and announcements. Each time the lights reflected off something shiny, they burned a brief, bright streak in the video tube.

"Come on, come on," Gabe said. "The elevator is farther over to the left."

"Okay, okay," Wolfe said. "This is not exactly a Maserati, you know?" The camera moved to the bottom of a staircase. The elevator doors came into view.

The camera zoomed in on the elevator call button. The robotic arm came into view from below. Wolfe succeeded in pressing the button on the second try. There was a smattering of applause from the techs.

The elevator doors opened. The screen showed a section of the elevator wall, then slowly turned around to face the front.

"What floor?" Wolfe said.

"Sixth."

They watched the screen. After two near misses, the robot arm pressed the button for the sixth floor.

When the doors opened, Gabe and the others saw the hallway and the rows of empty lab benches. The door to Gertrude's office appeared in the distance, growing gradually larger until it filled the screen.

"The lab is down the hall to the left," Gabe said.

Wolfe guided the device down the hall, stopping as it approached the door of the lab.

"Let's stop here for a reading," Wolfe said. "You can all relax. This'll take a few minutes." Wolfe let out a long breath, tugged at his ear, and moved to another computer keyboard.

It took nearly fifteen minutes. Wolfe kept turning dials, pressing buttons, and looking at the digital readout.

"Got it," he said. There was the sound of printing. A piece of paper the size of adding-machine tape came spooling out of a slot like a thin white tongue. Wolfe tore it off, looked at it, and stuck it under the spring of his clipboard.

"Well, what does it say?"

"Don't know if this is going to help or not," he said. "Either it's not working or there's not much there. Let's see if we can get that door open."

He operated the controls for the mechanical arm. Gabe watched the hand reach out toward the knob. It slipped off and went out of the picture.

The robot's third attempt was successful. The door opened a few inches. "Now let's see if I can put this baby into compound low," Wolfe said. His fingers darted over the keyboard. He inched the joystick forward. After what seemed an eternity, the edge of the door began to move across the screen.

"Come on, come on," Gabe said. "Is she in there or not?" He realized that he had been biting the insides of his cheeks.

"Easy, brother," Wolfe said gently. "This little devil takes its own sweet time."

The dark edge of the door passed across the screen, revealing a pattern of blurred squares.

"What the hell is that?" Hernandez said.

"Hold on to your britches." Wolfe adjusted the focus. They were looking at rows of small enclosures. The rats lay dead on the floors of their cages.

"Can we look around a little?" Gabe asked. It felt as if someone had taken a hammer to his heart.

"I'm trying, I'm trying," Wolfe said. The camera panned across the jumble on the lab bench, then zoomed in on two small gas canisters in a heavy metal case.

"There's your nerve gas," he said.

The camera did a 360-degree sweep of the room. It appeared to be empty.

"Wait a minute," Gabe said. "Go back. The fume hood."

Wolfe directed the lens to the far end of the room. The glass door of the fume hood was closed. The robot was directly across from the glass door. They were picking up a reflection from the lights.

"We're going to burn out the goddamn camera," Wolfe said. He turned off the flood lights. The fume hood, which had been painfully bright, now appeared solid black.

"Great. Much better," Gabe said.

"Hold your horses." Wolfe opened the shutter and brought the camera into focus. What had been a swirl of grays became a human figure sprawled on the work surface behind the closed door of the fume hood.

"It's Gertrude," Kate said. They all crowded around the monitor, trying to make sense of what they were seeing. Gertrude lay with her head on one outstretched arm. Her eyes were closed. Tears glistened on her cheeks. There was a dark pool of shiny liquid beneath her.

"*Jesus y María,*" Hernandez said.

Kate turned away from the screen. "That poor, sweet old lady," she said. She was crying softly now, resting her forehead against Gabe's back.

"What the hell is she doing inside the fume hood?" Wolfe asked.

Gabe was still studying the screen intently. "Wait a minute," he said. "She just moved."

"You're dreaming," Hernandez said.

"She did move," Wolfe said in a subdued voice. "What the hell's going on?"

Gabe grasped Wolfe's arm. "Don't you see? Somebody locked her in the room and opened the nerve gas. She got into the fume hood and turned on the oxygen," he said. "The positive pressure kept the nerve gas from getting in. Get those guys moving, will you? We've got to get her out of there."

"Baxter. Cavanaugh. Grab the fans. You're going up."

Kate crowded in beside them. "Oh, Gabe. She's alive. She's alive." Gabe felt her arms around him, the tightness in his throat, the warm tears running down his cheeks.

38

So how is she?" Kate asked. Gabe had just returned to his apartment from Gertrude's bedside at the University of California Hospital. Kate had just come back from a run.

"They've got her up in intensive care," he said. "They say she's pretty stable. Lew Watkins is taking care of her."

"What are her chances?" Kate asked, wiping her face with a towel.

"They're still trying to get the fluids out of her lungs. She's in a coma but she's got a fighting chance. It was a miracle she was able to get herself into the fume hood like that." Gabe poured kibble into the cat's dish. Princess attacked the food as if she hadn't eaten in a week.

"God. I would just die if anything happened to her," Kate said. She put a soft hand on his back.

Gabe nodded in agreement. "Can you imagine Ed sending somebody out to kill her?"

"Frankly, no," she said. "He's got to be much sicker than I ever realized. It's my fault. If I hadn't been out running when she called . . ."

Gabe put a hand on her arm. "Don't blame yourself," he said. "How was your run?"

"I felt guilty not being there at the hospital with you, but it was heaven," she said. "Running five miles when you're in shape to run twenty-six. Listen. Are you sure you're still up to riding along with me in the race tomorrow?"

"I wouldn't miss it," he said. "What are you going to need?"

"I've got my whole little routine. Eight squeeze bottles of water, one of Gatorade. One of defizzed Coke. Hot and cold coffee. A banana, a cookie, and a tube of Vaseline."

"What's that for?"

"Chafing under the arms. And remember—you can't touch me. Don't help me up if I fall. Don't even come close. I could be disqualified."

She went into his bathroom to shower. Gabe made a fresh pot of coffee, carried his cup into his office, sat down at his desk, and pushed the Play button on his answering machine. The fourth message was from Sheila:

"Gabe, I just heard something else that really worries me. The word at the company is that Kate has gone over to your side, so Santini has been instructed to go after her as well. I got the impression they might try something during the race tomorrow. Or afterward. I just overheard a few snatches of conversation so I'm not completely sure I've got this right, but I thought you'd want to know."

Gabe listened to the message several times. He removed the tape, replaced it with another, and put it in an envelope with Hernandez's name on it.

There was a thin red folder in his Urgent box. It was a packet from Lu Jean.

Dear Boss,
I've been playing around with that program you gave me and finally managed to uncover the rest of the text.

The guy who wrote it was a pretty slick programmer. Here's a printout of the stuff you didn't see before. Looks like he never finished the animation for this section. I'm including a copy of the disk. See you tomorrow.

—Lu Jean

The attached text read:

None of the animals experienced any adverse reactions during the preclinical tests. Phase 1 clinical trials likewise revealed no such difficulties. In Phase 2, a 39-year-old female developed a mild hypertensive crisis after receiving the drug while in the acute phase of a well-documented infection with Influenza A-182. Symptoms were controlled by routine treatment with no adverse outcome. There were no such reactions in Phase 3. However, theoretically, influenza or other viral illnesses could lead to stimulation of cytochrome P450, resulting in elevated levels of xanthosine reductase. Increased concentrations of this enzyme could change the qualitative or quantitative nature of Virazine clearance. Physicians should be warned of this possibility in the package insert.

Kate was sitting at the kitchen table, drying her hair. Gabe set Lu Jean's packet in front of her.

"What do you think of this?" he said.

She read through the note, sipping her coffee. "Sounds great," she said. "What the hell does it mean?"

"This must be what Howard was so worried about. One of the first patients in the clinical trials developed high blood pressure after taking Virazine. And she'd just had a case of this year's flu."

"The flu," Kate said. "Could that be the missing link?"

"Could be, darling," Gabe said. "It just could be."

At eleven that evening, Gabe and Kate were parked in Gabe's car, looking up at the lights in the pharmacology lab. They had been waiting and watching for more than an hour.

"So you think it's the flu changing the victims' liver enzymes?" Kate asked.

"It's got to be," Gabe said. "By the way, Monica Penny called again."

"The *60 Minutes* woman?"

"Yes. Apparently Monica's producer wasn't quite as impressed with the whole story as she was. He says they need a mechanism to explain what's happening."

"They're not going to run the piece if we can't find the mechanism?"

Gabe shrugged. "That's what she implied."

It was twenty after eleven when the fourth-floor windows finally went dark. They waited while a student with a backpack disappeared down the street, then used the stairs. They slipped into Gertrude's office without running into anyone.

Gertrude's lab was sealed off with yellow police tape, but her office was undisturbed. The papers were still stacked high in the row of baskets along the back of her desk.

"Here's where we start," Gabe said, pointing to the long row of lab notebooks in the bookshelf.

"My God," Kate said, astonished. "Dozens of them."

"This is just the last few months," Gabe said. "She's got a bunch more stored away somewhere."

"What are we looking for?" Kate said.

"Liver enzymes," Gabe said. "Influenza A-182. Cytochrome P450. Xanthosine reductase. Anything about changing pathways of drug breakdown. It could be a lab observation, some connection she made. Even something she read. From what she said over the phone, I'm sure she'd figured it out."

Gabe looked though the most recent lab books.

"Wait a minute," he said. "These go back a couple of months. The most recent ones are missing."

"Missing?"

"Yes. Damn it to hell. Whoever tried to kill her took her lab books too."

"Oh, Gabe."

"Wait a minute. Gertrude was very organized. She kept copies of everything. Look in the big bottom drawer of her desk."

They found photocopies of all the missing lab books. They were sorted into neat manila folders, the beginning and ending dates of each written neatly on the folder labels in Gertrude's small handwriting.

Gabe handed the folders to Kate. "You start with these," he said. "I'm going to look through her Must Read stack."

Two deep white-wire baskets stood on a raised shelf that ran along the back of the desk. The basket on the left contained correspondence, minutes of staff meetings, and various administrative reports. Each paper or group of papers had a yellow cover slip that indicated the date for follow-up or the person with whom it was to be discussed. Toward the middle of the basket Gabe found a single yellow page with a few notes. The cover slip read "Discuss w/Gabe A." The notes were as follows:

Possibilities:

no	1. Drug → Rx
no	2. Drug + MAO trigger → Rx
no	3. New strain + Drug → Rx
no	4. New strain + Drug + MAO trigger → Rx
no	5. Contamination
?	6. New strain + Factor X + MAO trigger → Rx
?	7. New strain + Drug + Factor X → Rx
?	8. Drug + Factor X + MAO trigger → Rx

"What is it?" Kate asked.

"A list of possible mechanisms," Gabe said. "I've seen her do it a thousand times. You list all the possible explanations for an observed phenomenon, then you investigate each one—beginning at the top of the list and working down." He shook his head. "I wish to hell I could talk to her for just five minutes."

"There's no chance she . . ."

"No," Gabe said. "She's stable but still unconscious. You find anything yet?"

Kate laughed and shook her head. "You got to give me a little time, babes," she said. "Nothing about Virazine or riboxyuridine or liver enzymes so far. But I've only gone back five days. She had a lot going: giving nerve gas to rats, purifying a synthetic mixture one of her students had come up with, giving rats some kind of a vaccination, developing a new assay for organophosphate in rat blood."

At twelve-thirty, Kate came and put her arms around his sholders. "I'm going to sack out on the couch. I've got a race tomorrow. Wake me when you're ready to go."

"Kate. That's crazy. I'll drive you home. You need to get a good night's sleep."

She shook her head. "I won't have any trouble sleeping," she said. "And I do want to be here with you. Really. I'll be fine."

Gabe sat at Gertrude's desk for several more hours, reading through her notebooks and papers and carefully rereading each of the victims' charts, while Kate slept on the couch. But look as he might, he was unable to come up with anything new.

It was nearly 3:00 A.M. when he shook Kate awake and they slipped away, down the stairs and out into the fog-kissed, pearl-black San Francisco morning.

39

In his dream, Gabe was being chased by monsters.

He was running across an urban nightscape during a thunderstorm. But the rain was sparkling confetti, and the buildings, the trees, even the sidewalks, were all canvas stage props.

The whole thing was taking place on the Lincoln

High School stage. The monsters were teenagers in creaking canvas costumes.

He sensed that the real monster was somewhere far out in the darkness, beyond the footlights, waiting and watching. He peered out past the stage lights, into the murky black silence, but he could see nothing.

"Gabe? What is it? Are you okay?" Kate had slipped her arms around his chest and laid her head against his shoulder.

"A bad dream," he said. He turned and slipped his arm around her. The bedside clock read 4:55 A.M.

Neither of them said anything for a long time. The dream hovered for a moment in the tangle of pillows and bedclothes, then suddenly vanished.

"Race day," he said. "You didn't get much sleep."

"I never do," she said. "I've been awake since four, visualizing. Why don't we get up and you can make us some coffee while I start stretching."

Kate slipped into a pair of shorts and a T-shirt. She put a blanket on the kitchen floor and started her usual series of stretches. "Do you know you were talking in your sleep?" she said.

"No." Gabe got down the jar of coffee beans and poured some into the grinder.

"You were yelling to me to watch out for something. I couldn't tell what." She lay on her stomach, bending her head and feet back until the soles of her feet brushed the crown of her head.

"Yeah?" He pushed the button and the grinder began to buzz, trembling in his hands like an angry living thing.

She nodded. "It scared me a little. You sounded so worried." She split her legs out to either side, leaned forward, and touched her chin to the gray tile of the kitchen floor. He put a paper filter in the machine and poured the fresh-ground coffee into it.

"Kate," he said. "Sheila called yesterday. She thinks that this guy Santini is after you as well. She got the impression they might try to do something during the race."

"Do something? Like what?"

"I don't know." He filled the coffeemaker with water, flipped the switch, and leaned back against the counter. "Did you tell any of the Kimberley people you were going to help me blow the whistle on Virazine?"

"I might have said something like that," she said.

"Who was it you told?"

She hesitated. "Ed." She sat with her legs out straight in front of her, bending at the waist until her head touched her knees, her fingers locked around the soles of her feet.

"You blew up at Ed?"

"Yes." She looked up angrily. "He accused me of spying on the company."

Gabe nodded and bit his lip. He drew a deep breath, looking down at the coffee dripping into the sparkling glass pot.

"Don't ask me not to run this race, Gabe. I want to beat Maritova just once before I die," she said. She lay flat on her back on the floor doing a series of pelvic tilts. "The weather is right. I know the course. I'm in good shape. This may be my best shot. Besides, you really think they'd try something during the race? With TV coverage and everything?"

Gabe shrugged. "They've done everything they've threatened before."

"I really think you're overreacting, sweetie." she said. "Paranoid, but sweet. Now you need to leave me alone for a while. I need to visualize my strategy one more time."

The starting line for the San Francisco Women's Marathon was in front of McLaren Lodge, near the corner of Stanyan and John F. Kennedy Drive. A dozen women in sleeping bags were huddled around a portable camp stove, drinking coffee from shiny metal cups. The scene was dominated by a three-story photo tower. A camera crew was milling around on top. A half-dozen photographers had taken up positions on the two lower levels.

Gabe parked under a streetlight across from McLaren Lodge and found Carlos Escobar on the lodge steps, whittling a soft piece of white cedar into what appeared to be an emaciated elephant. The elephant and the knife disappeared into his pockets in one smooth motion.

"Gabe. How you doing?"

"Fine. Thanks for coming."

"No problem." Carlos smiled, showing several gold teeth. He was a thin, restless man with a misshapen left shoulder.

Carlos and Gabe had played football together at Lincoln High. Carlos had been a shifty running back with great leg strength who could run over the middle all day, then kill you as a receiver coming out of the backfield. He was not particularly fast but had been nearly impossible to tackle. He had held the ball when Gabe kicked extra points. They had practiced together for hours.

"You bring your bike?" Gabe asked.

Carlos nodded. "Back in the bushes. You really think they going to try to whack your lady?"

Carlos had served with the special forces, working behind enemy lines in the early days of Vietnam. He had had a difficult time adjusting to civilian life. Just a few months earlier, Gabe had been a character witness at Carlos's assault trial. Carlos had broken a big biker's arm in a barroom brawl.

They walked back to the car and Gabe spread his San Francisco map out on the hood. He had marked out the course of the race in yellow Magic Marker.

"They start at the lodge, run west through the park for the first three miles, past the conservatory, behind the De Young Museum, past Stowe Lake, the buffalo pen, the golf course, and out to the windmill," Gabe said. He traced the course with his finger.

The forty-foot-high Murphy Windmill had been donated to the city by the Dutch government years ago. It stood a few hundred yards from the Great Highway, which ran along the ocean beach.

Carlos nodded, tracing the route with his finger. "South along the Great Highway to the zoo. They make a loop around Lake Merced and back to the windmill again. Then what?"

"They make a three-mile loop back into the park to make the distance come out right," Gabe said. The runners would pass the windmill a third time, heading north on the Great Highway, following Geary Boulevard, Twenty-fifth Avenue, and Lincoln Avenue on their way to the Golden Gate Bridge. They would cross the bridge in the two right-hand lanes.

"The finish line is at the little view spot on the Sausalito end of the bridge. They'll be able to film the winner coming across the line with the city across the water in the background."

Carlos shrugged. "Whatever," he said. "How long do we have?"

"It's five-forty now," Gabe said. "They start at eight. They're going to be closing the course. What do you say we go for a little drive?"

They got into Gabe's Volvo and drove slowly along the street leading into the park. They passed a team of three men in white painter's overalls. They were preparing to paint a wide white line across the road. Carlos raised an eyebrow.

"Mile markers," Gabe said. "They'll have a race worker with a microphone at each one, calling out the elapsed time."

Carlos nodded respectfully. "These ladies are pretty serious about all this."

The windmill was just over three miles from the starting line. Next to it was a second photo platform. Across from the tower they were setting up folding tables for the first water stop. In a little over two hours the runners would come thundering past, expecting to have five thousand paper cups of water ready and waiting. Behind the tables were five white trucks from the Alhambra Water Company. A shivering young man in a 49ers cap was driving a heavily loaded forklift down a steep ramp from the back of a flatbed truck.

"You know," Carlos said. "I wanted to do somebody, I'd probably set up right here."

"Here?" Gabe said. "Nah. Too many spectators."

"That's what you want, man. Lots of confusion. Nobody's going to know what happened at first. Bop. You do it. The crowd makes it easy to slip away."

They followed the Great Highway south. It was a rather undistinguished four-lane road built along the top of a long seawall. The offshore breeze blew the sand across the southbound lane. They passed the zoo, took a left at Skyline Boulevard, and stopped at Lake Merced. "The runners follow the footpath through the golf course around the lake," Gabe said.

Carlos shook his head and smiled. "Now, your Cong would *love* this setup, but you're most likely going to be dealing with some city cat. A city kid would never pick a place like this. They like to be able to do the deed and disappear into a crowd."

They returned to the windmill, turned right into the park, and made the three-mile loop up South Drive, around the Arboretum, and back along Lincoln Way, the park's southern border. As they passed the windmill for the third time, Carlos punched Gabe on the shoulder. "This is the place, man," he said. "They come by here three times. You use the first two to check out the situation, make your game plan. Then, the third time you go for it."

They drove north past the Cliff House, took a right on Geary, followed it to Twenty-fifth Avenue, turned north on Twenty-fifth, drove into the Presidio, and followed Lincoln Avenue through the army base to the Golden Gate Bridge. The east lane of the bridge was blocked off by a mile-long row of orange, cone-shaped traffic markers. They drove slowly past the scenic area on the Sausalito side.

A policeman in a reflective vest was waving traffic away from the view spot. Gabe pulled over and joined a line of rubberneckers parked on the freeway shoulder.

"Stay here a minute, buddy," Gabe said. "I want to check this out."

He made a quick circuit around the view spot. A large digital race clock stood on one side of the finish line, the third photo tower on the other. Behind the line were four trucks with cherry pickers that would maneuver photographers into position for shots of the winners coming across the finish line.

NBC had set up a temporary studio in a complex of trailers. He could see the sportscasters' desk behind a big plate glass window, providing a background of the Golden Gate and the city across the Bay.

"Funny setup," Carlos said, as Gabe got back into the car.

"The media like it," Gabe said. "It's hard to cover a marathon. This way they can watch the start, jump on a bus to the windmill, watch the leaders go by three times, then bus out here for the finish.

"So you wouldn't do it here?" Gabe asked.

Carlos shook his head. "No way, man. Impossible to get out. And the whole place is crawling with cops. I can promise you this: you get your girl on the bridge, she's home free."

"So it's got to be the woods, the windmill, or somewhere in the park?" Gabe said.

Carlos nodded. "Or nowhere at all."

"That's always a possibility," Gabe said.

40

Gabe loaded the bottles of hot and cold coffee, the water bottles, and the defizzed Coke into the baskets of his bike. He carried it out to the sidewalk and sat on the steps, reading the sports section until Kate came out.

She seemed to glow against the soft light of the morning fog, strong and vulnerable and acutely alive. She wore a rose-colored warmup suit over her white nylon racing outfit.

"What does the paper say?" She bent forward to retie a shoelace.

"Maritova's the champion," Gabe said. "You're our dark horse hometown favorite. They've got your picture."

"Oh, God. The one from Seattle with my hair all plastered to my head. And there's Katrina with her perfect little golden braid. Why can't *I* look like that?"

She jogged beside him as he rode his bike slowly toward the park. "Did you find anything else last night? After I went to sleep?"

Gabe shook his head. "I went back through the victims' medical records. As far as I can tell, none of them had the flu," he said. "Not a single one. So much for our great lead from Howard."

"So Factor X is not the flu," she said.

"Apparently not."

They crossed Stanyan Street and joined the surging stream of humanity that was pushing into the park. There were already a thousand women within a block of the starting line. The big race clock read 7:07.

It was supposed to be one of the largest women's marathons ever. There would be more than five thousand competitors from all over the world. Most of them were already there—stretching, jogging, meditating, or waiting in long lines at the bright orange Sani-Cans—thousands of healthy women bathed in the soft red light of the morning sky. Kate found an empty bit of lawn, put down her beach towel, and went into another stretching routine. Gabe leaned his bike against a tree and hunkered down beside her.

"So listen," he said. "Before the media folks find you. I have a little surprise."

She looked up suspiciously, pausing in the middle

of a hurdler's straddle stretch. "I don't much like surprises on race days."

Gabe took a tiny pair of earphones out of his pocket. "Lu Jean brought these back from an electronics trade show," he said. "It's an ultralight walkie-talkie. It weighs less than an ounce."

"Gabe, I don't need *any* extra weight."

"You won't even notice. I promise."

"Goddammit. Why do you have to pull a stunt like this at the last minute?"

"Look, Kate. This could be a real professional job, especially after what happened to Gertrude. And Howard." He held the earphones out to her. "They'll let me communicate with you. And you with me. I've checked the rules. It's perfectly legal. Here's the mike. You flip it down like this."

She took them unwillingly, weighing them in her hand. "But what *good* are they going to do? Really— what's the point?"

"If I see anything I can let you know. And if *you* need anything or have any trouble you can talk to *me*."

She took the headphones and put them on, flipping the mike down and back up again. "I'll do it on one condition," she said. "If I feel like they're slowing me down, I'm going to dump 'em."

"Hey, Gabe, what're you doing, poaching on our territory?" It was Thad Murray, the Channel 7 sports reporter. The bearded cameraman balanced a dented minicam on his shoulder.

"Hey, Thad. No, she's all yours."

"Thanks." He turned to Kate. "So. Dr. Reiley. Can we talk to you for a minute?"

Gabe took the opportunity to walk over to the starting line. He found himself surrounded by eager, excited women of all ages, from young girls to lithe grandmas, dressed in T-shirts and running silks in a hundred bright colors. He walked through a sea of nylon-clad womanhood. They were filling cups from Thermos bottles, receiving final instructions, exchanging hugs and kisses with coaches, parents, children, husbands, lovers. They filled the whole east end of the park and spilled out onto the streets, blocking traffic.

After Kate finished with the press, Gabe got her to put on the headphones and rode up the street to do a sound check. A hundred yards away he stopped, straddled his bike, and whispered into the mike: "You've got a cute ass. If you can hear me, shake it." He could see her reach up to pull the microphone down.

"Why, *Dr. Austin*," she said in her best shocked, schoolmarm voice. "How *terribly* unprofessional." But she did a little wiggle just the same.

It wasn't until the race announcer called the seeded runners to the starting line that Gabe saw Katrina Maritova. She was a tall, handsome woman, her long blond hair in a single braid. She wore light-blue silks. Her running shoes were freshly whitened. She looked more like a Nordic goddess than a marathon runner. Kate, a head shorter, looked like a child beside her.

The tension mounted as the announcer counted down the last minutes. Gabe rode on ahead, pulled up on a little rise, and took out his binoculars. Kate and Maritova stood shoulder to shoulder in the middle of the starting line.

As the announcer began counting off the final seconds, three motorcycle policemen and the big blue open-backed moving van that housed the NBC camera crew pulled into place.

Gabe saw a puff of smoke and a moment later heard the report of the starter's gun. The spectators let out a cheer and the mob of women began to move forward. Kate and Maritova were in front, right behind the flashing blue lights of the police motorcycles.

41

Gabe rode along a hundred yards ahead of the police escort. The spectators kept spilling over into the street to get a view of the leaders, and he had to pick his way carefully through the crowd.

He rode ahead to the first-mile mark and pulled up beside the race official who was preparing to call out the one-mile times over his bullhorn. He looked back with his binoculars and saw that two thin teenagers in UC–Berkeley T-shirts were ahead, sprinting flat-out, playing for the cameras, already beginning to wilt. Katrina was in third place, twenty yards behind them. Kate was at her shoulder. Her face was calm and quiet and she was running gracefully and without apparent effort.

Gabe flipped down the mike. "You're looking absolutely beautiful, kiddo," he said. Her head jerked up. He could see her looking around.

"I'm up ahead of you, on the right, just past the one-mile mark. Let me know if you need anything." She spotted him and gestured toward her mouth with her thumb.

Both Kate and Maritova finished the first mile in 5:15, right on their usual pace. Gabe pulled ahead of the pack and stayed there until the college girls had staggered off to the side. He then dropped back beside Kate and tossed her a water bottle, being careful not to touch her. She squirted it into her mouth, then tossed it back.

By the time the windmill came into view Kate was still at Maritova's shoulder. Their nearest competitors were now more than a hundred yards behind. Gabe kept his bike twenty yards ahead of the police motorcycles. He had wired one earphone to an FM scanner and was listening to the audio of the race coverage on the local NBC-TV station.

Much of the same crowd that had been at the start now lined the roadway on either side of the windmill. As they neared the water station, Maritova slowed down to pick up a drink. Kate took the opportunity to step up her pace. She swung around the taller woman and began to pull away. There was a surprised murmur on all sides, then the crowd burst into applause. The photographers in the tower went into action, the sound of their motor drives buzzing like a hundred tiny submachine guns. The NBC commentator sounded excited for the first time all day.

Gabe glanced across at the press platform and felt his blood run cold. Chip Downey was standing on the grass, leaning back against one of the corner pillars, arms crossed, a cigarette in his mouth, his mirrored glasses covering his eyes. When he saw Gabe his mouth tightened and he turned away, ducking out of sight behind the water truck.

Gabe pulled over, got out his binoculars, and looked back at the tower. An army of photographers jammed each of the three levels. Others occupied the lower limbs of trees, the tops of cars, and the back of the empty water truck. He couldn't see Downey or anything else out of the ordinary.

Gabe switched the walkie-talkie to another frequency.

"Carlos. You there?"

"Loud and clear, man. Hey, that lady of yours sure got some class. You see her pull away from that German bitch?"

"Yeah. Where are you?"

"Across from the tower."

"Good man. Look, you see the big guy in the blue jacket and the silver shades? He just ducked behind the water truck?"

"I see him."

"Good. Keep an eye on him. His name is Downey and he's one of the company guys. Watch him like a hawk. Look for any sign of a gun. And watch the other photographers."

"Roger wilco."

"Any cops around there?"

"Yeah, a couple on horses. They've been circulating."

"Okay. See if you can get close to our man before the runners come back. You see anything funny, knock him down and sit on him. Let's not take any chances."

Gabe caught up with Kate just before she reached the ocean. She was setting the pace now, with Maritova trailing by twenty yards. As Gabe came up alongside Kate she allowed herself a faint smile, lifted one arm, and pointed up under it. Gabe tossed her the tube of Vaseline and she rubbed some under each arm. Maritova took the opportunity to sprint forward.

They battled back and forth for the lead. Maritova ended up a few steps in front. Kate tossed back the tube, winked, and tucked in behind her, keeping a bit to the left to let the taller woman break the cool, steady breeze coming in from the ocean. The announcer reminded his audience for the dozenth time that Kate had the best finishing kick in the field. Maritova would need to build up a substantial lead going onto the bridge if she hoped to win. Gabe trailed along behind until Kate asked for another drink, tossed her a bottle, then stood up on his pedals and went ahead to check the running trail around Lake Merced.

There was virtually no one there. As he rode by the police pistol range he heard occasional sounds of gunfire, like a few leftover grains of popcorn in a hot pan. He searched the trees and bushes carefully but saw nothing except two golfers beating the bushes for a lost ball.

As they finished the loop around the lake and came back to the Great Highway, Maritova made her move. Starting at the 12-mile mark, she lengthened her stride, picked up the pace, and slowly began to pull away.

The announcer took that opportunity to put on a clip from the interview Kate had given them that morning. "My strategy's no secret," she said in that matter-of-fact way of hers. "Katrina will try to build up a big lead between twelve and twenty miles. That's her strongest part of the race. It's the time I usually slow down. I'm going to stay with her as best I can. If I'm within striking distance at twenty miles, I'll have a good chance to win the race."

By the time they were halfway along the beach Gabe saw that Maritova was ahead by 150 yards and was increasing her lead. Her light-blue figure with the tossing braid was growing smaller and smaller in the distance. Kate was taking a lot of fluid, alternating coffee and water. Gabe began to worry that she was drinking too much.

By the time they reached the park again Maritova

had increased her lead to 250 yards. Gabe pulled ahead to check out the situation around the windmill. He peddled past Katrina and the camera truck and switched the walkie-talkie back to Carlos's channel.

"We're three-quarters of a mile away," Gabe said. "What's our friend doing?"

"Not much. Just hanging around smoking."

"Anybody with him?"

"Not that I've seen."

"Keep an eye on him."

"I'm in his hip pocket."

Gabe stopped short of the windmill, took out his binoculars, and scanned the tower, paying close attention to the photographers. He didn't see anything unusual. Perhaps he *was* imagining things. Maybe Downey was just an avid sports fan.

The flashing blue lights were coming up fast behind him. He stopped across from the tower and watched Katrina come by, slowing down for the water stop. As she passed in front of him he pressed the button on his stopwatch. One minute and ten seconds later Kate came past.

Kate's voice in his ear surprised him: "How far ahead is she?"

"A minute ten," he said.

"Damn." He could hear her breathing hard.

"Drink?"

"Yes. The Coke."

He caught up with her and tossed her the bottle. She promptly dropped it. He went back, picked it up, and threw it to her again. Kate looked tired now, her skin pulled tightly over her cheekbones. He saw traces of weariness and discouragement in her face.

There was a good crowd all the way through the park. As they passed mile 18 at Twenty-eighth Street, the race official told him that Maritova was one minute twenty seconds ahead. Four hundred yards. An almost insurmountable lead. She had been out of Gabe's sight ever since the leaders left the Great Highway.

He called Carlos once again. "Final time, buddy. Still got our man?"

"Sure do. He looks a little nervous. He just finished his tenth— Wait a minute. He's moving. Away from the road."

"Stay with him."

"All right. I'll have to leave my bike."

"Leave it."

Gabe watched as Carlos leaned his bike against a tree and moved out of sight behind a grove of trees.

"He's going back into the bushes," Carlos said.

"Stay with him."

"Shit. He's taking a piss."

Gabe raced ahead of Maritova again. She looked somewhat fatigued but still very much in control, very confident. Gabe pulled over behind the water stop and scanned the tower with his binoculars as the photographers watched the leader go past. Maritova paused briefly at the water stop. Almost as an afterthought, Gabe decided to check out the half-dozen photographers who had set up on the flatbed truck.

He had to look twice to make sure that he had really seen a rifle barrel taped to the side of one of the long telephoto lenses. A slight, dark figure in a green hooded sweatshirt was looking through the telephoto sight at the empty road. He had set up his tripod on the flatbed, right next to the cab of the truck. Gabe looked back and saw Kate coming up quickly. She was doing her best to narrow the gap.

He was a good thirty yards from the truck. He jumped onto his bike and began pedaling furiously across the road. As he passed the tower he was aware of a figure running toward him. It was Downey. He held a thick length of two-by-four in his hands. Before Gabe could avoid him he jammed it hard into his rear spokes. Gabe heard the crunch of twisted metal. The road came up and hit him. He rolled over and over. Then he was lying on his back, the breath knocked out of him. He looked up and saw an angry race official running toward him.

Gabe made himself get up. His forehead was cut and there was blood running into his eyes. The back wheel of his bike was a tangle of broken spokes. The race official was pulling him away from the road. Gabe saw that he was not going to be able to get to Kate.

He turned and ran toward the truck, slipping on the soggy grass. Kate was nearly opposite the tower now. He could see the gunman sighting along the rifle, tracking the point where she would pass. The crowd was in a frenzy. No one would notice the sound of a shot.

Gabe hit the ramp at the back of the truck sprinting at full speed. His chest was heaving and he felt a terrible moment of light-headedness. Then his mouth opened and a horrible, angry sound came out. The other photographers started and pulled away, one even jumping off the truck, making it easier for Gabe to bull his way through.

He had never run so fast in his life. Cameras and tripods went flying. He crashed into the gunman, slapping the barrel of the rifle upward with his right hand just as it went off.

Gabe fell on top of the gunman and both went down against the cold metal of the cab, the tripod crashing on top of them. The sound of the shot was still ringing in Gabe's ears.

The hooded figure was small but very strong. Gabe

tried to grasp his throat, but the gunman grabbed Gabe's arm and twisted it behind him. He caught Gabe in the throat with an open-handed karate blow, then hit him hard in the solar plexus.

By the time Gabe was able to sit up, the hooded figure had disappeared. Gabe had not seen his face.

There was a turmoil of angry voices. Then the crowd began to realize what Gabe had done. There were cheers. People were calling for the police. Then Carlos was kneeling beside him.

"Shit, man. I really screwed up. You all right?"

"I'm fine. Is Kate . . ."

"She's okay, man. I don't think she even noticed. You got to that son of a bitch just in time. These bastards must have spotted me. They really set me up."

Gabe dragged himself to his feet. The horizon was tilting back and forth. "Where's Downey?" he asked.

"I've got him hogtied. He's not going anywhere for a while."

"Good man. You stay here and deal with the cops. Tell them to call Hernandez in Homicide. I'm taking your bike.

"Sure, go for it. Looks like your radio survived. You sure you're okay?"

There was a confused smattering of applause as Gabe transferred his gear into the basket of Carlos's trail bike. He looked at his watch. The whole affair had taken less than three minutes.

42

Gabe rode Carlos's bike overland across the park to Fulton Street and headed north on Forty-seventh. He reached Geary Boulevard just ahead of the police escort.

Maritova still appeared totally in control. Kate was now nearly 500 yards behind. She looked pale and frazzled. He pulled over and rode beside her. When she saw him she made an exasperated face.

"Gabe. What *was* all that? My God, you're bleeding."

"I took a little spill. Everything's fine. You're going to win, baby. You need a drink?"

"Yes, maybe just one more. How far back am I?"

He tossed her the defizzed Coke. "About a minute and a half," he lied.

"It's more than that," she said. Gray clouds had moved over the sun. It was getting colder.

"You're beautiful," he said. "You're going to win, babes. Time for the famous Reiley kick."

"I don't know how much of a kick I've got left," she said. "I'm feeling pretty tired."

"You're going to do it," he said. "Last five miles coming up. You're in your territory now." His legs were getting tired from the short pedal stroke. The next mile was number 21, at Sutro Park. He distracted her so she wouldn't hear the time as they crossed the mile marker. She had fallen even farther behind.

"Maritova's slowing down," he lied again. "You just picked up half a minute."

"Really? That's great. I was really afraid something had happened to you."

"I'm fine," he said. "You can still do it. You're wonderful. And I love you."

She smiled. He thought he could see her lengthen her stride a bit.

"I'm going to see if I can send you a little good energy."

He'd been hooking the alligator clips from Carlos's Walkman onto the leads of his walkie-talkie transmitter. He inserted a cassette tape from his pocket, checked the whole jury-rigged apparatus carefully, and pushed the Play button.

The music was loud in his ears as Carly Simon sang that she was born to run, to be ahead of the rest, and that all she ever wanted was to do her best. It was Kate's theme song, the one she played on her Walkman during her tough training runs. As he rode alongside he saw tears come into her eyes. She pressed her lips together, gave him a rueful smile, and began to pour it on.

The leaders turned north on Twenty-fifth Street. There was more of a crowd here, many of them with radios and portable TVs. They began applauding as soon as Kate turned the corner, calling out to her, urging her on.

"Go for it, Katie! You can do it."

"Go get 'em, Doc!"

"We're pulling for you, Kate. Don't give up!"

"Come on, hometown girl!"

On the corner of Twenty-fifth and California, a ten-year-old girl held up a hand-printed sign:

When I grow up,
I want to be like
Kate Reiley

Kate gained ground steadily all the way through the Presidio. They passed the 25-mile mark and looped under Doyle Drive. As they came out on the right-hand lane of the Golden Gate Bridge, Maritova's bouncing blond braid came into view.

She was slowing badly. She glanced back fearfully at Kate, as if realizing that she had gone out a little too fast. Her pace was uneven. She appeared winded and spent.

The wind was cold from the ocean. Kate was not talking now. She was not smiling. She was running, using every bit of her energy and concentration.

When the crowd on the bridge saw that Kate was gaining ground, they went crazy. Kate increased her pace, going up on her toes in a final sprint for the finish line a mile away, her heels grazing her buttocks with each step, her arms pumping as if she were doing the hundred-yard dash.

The announcer was so excited he was having trouble controlling himself. "It's the famous Reiley kick. And Maritova is definitely fading. Reiley is only thirty yards behind. Twenty-five. Twenty. Watch out. Here she comes."

Gabe slackened his pace, letting himself drop behind. She was on the bridge. There was nothing more he could do.

As they reached the middle of the span, Kate was only ten yards behind. Then she seemed to stumble. For a terrible moment Gabe suspected that there might be another gunman on the bridge. Katrina seemed to be pulling ahead. But Kate had not given up. She steadied her stride and went up on her toes again, running downhill now, on the Marin side of the bridge.

She caught Maritova at the north tower. The German, clearly spent, struggled to keep up. Her stride was choppy, and she gasped audibly with each breath.

Kate passed her as if she were standing still. Then Kate began to really pour it on, running now not for victory or for personal glory but for the very joy of it.

She ran those last two hundred yards with a grave, regal quality that came across as clearly to the millions watching on television as it did to the wildly cheering crowd. For many days thereafter, the sports columnists raved about "The Kick." There were few athletes who could reach down into themselves and pull out the performance that Kate Reiley put on in that last mile. Maritova was a valiant champion. But on that Sunday afternoon it was the hometown favorite, Kate Reiley, who had led them all—runners and spectators alike—into a state of perfect grace.

43

"Congratulations," Monica Penny said to Kate. "That was quite a finish. Maybe we can work it into the program." They were sitting in Gabe's Volvo, parked across the street from Gertrude's pharmacology lab, waiting for the last graduate student to go home.

"If there *is* a program," Kate said.

"There's going to be a program if I have to wring my senior producer's neck." Monica had called them at Gabe's apartment that afternoon. The senior producer at "60 Minutes" had selected the Virazine piece as a "probable" for the following Sunday, and she had received authorization to begin videotaping.

She had brought along Bernie Swain, a local freelance camera and sound man, a nervous little longhaired guy who looked like a pimply Buster Keaton. Bernie's equipment was in the trunk.

"Your producer still doesn't sound too sure," Kate said.

"Trust me," Monica said. "It's going to happen. Anything new on your friend Gertrude?"

"Still the same—stable but unconscious," Gabe

said. "But we've figured out the mechanism. You'll have it on tape tonight."

The three of them stared at him in silence.

"Gabe?" Kate said. "Are you kidding?"

"So tell us," Monica said.

Gabe smiled. "I'll do it on camera," he said. "You can get it all on tape."

Monica nodded. "Smart," she said. "Now if we can just get these characters to go home."

"It's all sounds pretty mysterious to me," Bernie said, shaking his head. "So how come I never met you before?" He had a voice that started somewhere beneath his adenoids and echoed up through his sinuses.

"I usually work Chicago and the East Coast," Monica said. "The New York office told me I should call you. Here, have something to eat." She pushed the white McDonald's bag over to his side of the seat.

Kate leaned across the emergency brake and touched Gabe's arm. "So when did you figure it out?"

Gabe smiled and took her hand. "This afternoon. After the race. While you were out soaking in the hot tub."

"You heard something new?"

"Nope. I was lying down, thinking. Something just clicked. I got on the phone and did some checking. It was all so obvious."

It was half an hour later when the lab windows finally went dark. They waited a few moments, then made their way through the front door and down to the animal room.

"This place smells like the dung house at the circus," Bernie said.

"Bernie. Please," Monica ordered. "Just keep filming."

Gabe located the rats they wanted. He and Kate loaded the cages on a cart. They entered Gertrude's lab without incident. Bernie followed, taping everything.

Kate lowered the blinds. Bernie set up his lights and camera and taped Gabe as he used a small syringe to administer oral doses of the Virazine solution to the rats.

"Okay, we're rolling," Monica said. "So tell us—how did you figure it out?"

"From the things we found in her office," Gabe said. "There's a whole section in her lab notebook about vaccinating a group of rats with a killed culture of Influenza A-182."

"But I thought the nerve gas killed them all," Kate said.

Gabe smiled. "You don't know Gertrude. She always keeps a backup."

"So she vaccinated some rats," Monica said. "How do you know that's connected to Virazine?"

"Can you think of any other reason to give last year's flu shot to a rat? Besides, there was a paper on her desk about the transformation of liver enzymes that resulted from the same flu vaccine."

Monica shook her head. "But I thought none of the victims had had the flu."

"Right," Gabe said. "That was the tipoff. *None* of the victims had had the flu. It wasn't the flu that increased their liver enzymes. It was the Influenza A-182 flu shot."

"They'd all had flu shots?" Kate said.

Gabe nodded. "Yep. I checked them out today. Lindsey had hers at San Francisco State. Blumberg had been to the Orient. He got his at the Public

Health Service. Juan Rodriguez had his at the University school. Hattie Mae Davis got it at work. And I had to do a lot of calling on the San Francisco General patients, but they had all gotten one, too."

"And these rats have all had the same flu shot?" Monica asked.

"That's right."

"And now you're giving them Virazine and a tyramine trigger."

"You got it."

"All ready?" Kate asked.

Gabe nodded. "I hope they're hungry. Want to do the honors?"

"My pleasure," Kate said. Bernie rolled the camera as Kate unwrapped the Camembert cheese and placed it in the center of the cage.

Bernie wrinkled his nose. "That stuff would kill anything," he said.

The rats sniffed at the cheese, then began nibbling.

"How long's this going to take?" Monica asked.

Gabe shook his head. "I'm not sure."

Kate held a floodlight while Bernie took some close-ups of individual rats gnawing at the gradually shrinking wheel of cheese.

"So tell us what's going to happen," Monica said. "Make it real simple."

Gabe moved to the blackboard. "Let's say Virazine gets broken down into molecules A and B, which are both harmless." He drew two circles, labeling them A and B. "No problem. But let's say the flu shot changes your liver enzymes. So now the drug gets broken down into molecules X and Y. Molecule Y is harmless but molecule X is deadly."

"Then everybody who had the flu shot and took Virazine would get elevated blood pressure, even though *nobody* reacted before the flu shot came out,'' Monica said.

"Not quite." Gabe shook his head. "That would be a nice simple two-stage interaction. But everyone who gets the flu shot and takes Virazine *doesn't* get sick. So we must be dealing with something even more complicated—a *three*-stage interaction."

"Don't use such big words," Monica said. "You've got to keep it very simple."

"All right," Gabe said. "How about this: Step one is the flu shot. That's like loading the gun. Step two is the drug. That's like pulling back the hammer."

"But something still has to pull the trigger. Right?"

"Right. That's what Gertrude called Factor X."

"So what is it?"

Gabe pointed down at the rats' cage. "It's sitting right there in front of us."

"What?"

"The cheese. Aged, smelly cheese is full of an amino-acidlike compound called tyramine. A lot of other foods have it too: Pickled herring. Beer. And Chianti wine. Avocados. Chicken livers. Pâté. Some kinds of sausages. Fava beans. And there are a bunch of drugs that can produce a very similar reaction."

"And all the victims ate one of these triggers?"

"Right." Gabe nodded. "Lindsey Troutman ate a big bowl of leftover guacamole. Blumberg ate a big pizza with pepperoni and mozzarella. Juan Rodriguez ate a sausage sandwich. Hattie Mae Davis had just eaten a fava-bean casserole at a potluck. And of the San Francisco General patients, one took a cold remedy, one took diet pills, and one drank a whole bottle of Chianti."

"So let me get this straight," Monica said. "If somebody had the flu shot, took Virazine, and ate one of these foods or drugs . . ."

"Hey, you guys, come look." Kate's voice was

excited. Bernie turned the camera, directing the bright lights to the cage on the floor.

Gabe and Monica crowded in behind them, peering down at the cage. One of the rats had begun to twitch. Another began to tremble. As they watched, several others began to show signs of distress. The room was echoing with a squeaking chorus.

"My God," Kate said. "They're dying. They're really dying." Several of the rats were now lying on their sides on the floor of the cage, writhing in pain.

"Bernie, I want some pans from the rats to Gabe and Kate and back. Give me half a dozen of them." As the camera rolled, the rats began to go into convulsions. Within twenty minutes they were all either comatose or dead.

Kate looked up at Gabe, her eyes shining. "Well," she said softly, slipping her arms around him. "A little grisly, but I guess you did it. Congratulations, sweetie. You figured it out after all."

44

Kate peered ahead into the thick fog that billowed across the Golden Gate Bridge, slowing the evening northbound rush hour to a crawl. She had been subdued and silent all day. They had spent the day at Gabe's apartment, watching the tapes from the previous evening, shooting a few follow-up questions, and plotting their strategy. A little after noon Gabe had received an anonymous faxed message: The hidden ADRs had been moved to a file in the flea-collar production area.

Gabe turned to Kate. "You know where that is?"

Kate looked across at him uneasily. "Yes. It's in the nerve gas area. You have to wear a filtration suit to get in there."

The fax had been unsigned and there had been none of the usual identifying names or numbers, just a short, typed message. Gabe had gone into the other room, dug into his files, and brought back a packet of material he had received from Sheila. Her cover note was in the same typeface.

Kate shrugged. "Half the word processors at the company look like that," she said. "It could be anybody. It could be the person who sent me the original ADRs."

"There's one other possibility," Gabe said.

"What's that?" Monica asked.

"It's almost impossible to trace a fax," Gabe said. "This could be some kind of a trap."

Kate shook her head. "If it is, Monica and Bernie are the best protection we could have. No one would be nuts enough to try anything with a *60 Minutes* crew around."

They were driving Kate's Saab—it had a Kimberley parking sticker and would be less conspicuous. The back deck and most of the rear seat were crammed full of Bernie's equipment. Bernie and Monica were crowded into a corner. Bernie was fidgeting in the seat, his eyes darting around nervously. Monica shook her head and turned to him.

"What's eating you?" she snapped.

"I've been shot at twice before," Bernie said. "I don't like it."

"Bernie, look. Calm down. Get this out of my way, will you? I need a little room." Bernie took the blue metal box from the floor at her feet and held it tightly in his lap. Monica leaned forward and put a hand on Kate's arm. "You really think you can get us in?"

Kate nodded. "Unless they've changed the access to the heating tunnel."

"You see?" Monica said, patting Bernie on the shoulder. "The worst that can happen is we don't make it."

"Wrong," Bernie moaned. "The worst that can happen is I wind up with a security guard's slug in my gut."

"I'll bet they don't even carry guns," Monica said. "Kate? Am I right?"

"Just the supervisors," Kate said.

Gabe sensed Monica's rising excitement, like a hunter on the way to the kill. Her eyes were bright, and she had repeatedly licked off and renewed her lipstick. Gabe leaned forward in his seat, putting fresh batteries into the four pocket flashlights he had picked up at the pharmacy.

Monica asked Kate, "How're you going to get us in?"

Kate smiled. "Someone once bet Howard that he couldn't find a way into the building without going through security. It took him less than a day."

It was just after six-thirty when they drove into the Kimberley parking garage. Kate drove up the ramp to the third floor and pulled into a parking place against the far wall.

"Here we are," she said. "There's our door right there."

"That thing?" Gabe asked. A waist-high metal plate was set into the dingy cinderblock wall.

"That's it," Kate said.

"It's got to be locked," Gabe said.

"It's not." Kate shook her head, her eyes wide. "There are just a couple of screws you can turn with a coin."

"Hold it," Gabe said. "Don't get out. Sit still." A man came out of the elevator at the other end of the third level. He got into his car and drove away without looking in their direction. There were no other cars within view.

"Okay," Kate said. "Let's go." They all got out of the car. Kate showed Gabe how the turnscrews worked. As he loosened the final screw the metal door came free in his hands.

"No sweat," he said, leaning it against the wall. He switched on his flashlight and pointed it inside. A damp passageway led into the darkness.

"God, there must be rats," Bernie said. "And it's so narrow. How am I going to carry all my stuff?"

"Relax, we'll help you," Monica smiled a manic smile, her white teeth bright in the rays of their flashlights. "Damn. Into the bowels of darkness, huh?"

They piled the camera gear inside, then climbed in after it. Kate pulled the metal plate into place behind them and the daylight disappeared.

The passageway was cramped, steamy, and monotonous. Gabe followed behind the others, weighed down with two heavy boxes of camera equipment. Five minutes later they stepped through a similar hatch and found themselves in a janitor's closet. Gabe checked his watch. It was five minutes to seven. They were on the lower floor, just down the hallway from Howard's lab.

"All right, there should be no problem from here on," Kate said. "I'm going to take you straight through to the production area."

She led them down the hallway to the elevator. They rode up one floor and walked down another long hall to the production area, passing a row of open offices where two cleaning women called back and forth to each other.

Kate used her card to open the automatic doors. They stepped through into the bright, deserted corridor.

"Is there a watchman or what?" Monica said.

"He won't be back for another hour," Kate said.

They started down the corridor. Long windows on each side of the hallway looked in on the sterile work areas. The production equipment stood silent, the shiny metal belts, vats, and machines clean and gleaming.

"Any of these the machines you use to make Virazine?" Monica asked.

"Right over there," Kate said.

"Okay. We can use a quick shot of that," Monica said. "Zoom in slowly."

Bernie set up a tripod and began taping the silent machinery. Monica walked up the hallway, her hands behind her back. Gabe heard her gasp, and then saw her running back toward them, holding a finger to her lips and waving frantically.

"Ssssshh. It's the guard. I don't think he saw me."

They hurried along the corridor as quickly and quietly as they could. At the far end Gabe saw the glass doors with the sign: DANGER. NERVE GAS.

"Where are these files?" Monica whispered.

"In there." Kate pointed in through the glass doors at the moving belt in the flea collar production area.

They followed Kate into an antechamber where a row of white filtration suits hung on chrome hooks. Monica made a palms-down gesture and they all dropped to the floor.

They lay quietly for several minutes. At last Kate rose on one knee.

"It's clear," she said. "I'll need to put on a suit to get into the room where the records are."

Monica nodded. "Let's all go," she said.

"No," Kate said. "It's too dangerous. I'll go in by myself and bring them back. You can tape it through the window."

"I'll go for that," Bernie said. "I'm really not too fond . . ."

"We'll all suit up and go in," Monica said. "Trust me. This is going to make a great shot."

Kate shook her head. "I'm really not willing to put anybody else at risk," she said. "We can get all the footage you want from out—"

"Put on the suits. Please. All of you," Monica urged. There was controlled fury in her face. "This is going to be the crucial scene in the whole piece. It'll be great, believe me."

"I'm sorry, Monica," Kate said. "I'm just not willing to expose—"

She stopped suddenly, her face frozen. Gabe turned and saw that Monica was pointing a small black automatic at Kate's chest. She swiveled to point it at him.

"No more back talk," Monica said, her voice calm and authoritative. "Get into those suits."

"Monica?" Bernie asked. "What the hell is this?"

She turned the gun on him. "You want to give me an excuse? Go ahead. Say one more word, you disgusting little insect."

"Gabe . . ." Kate held the billowing plastic suit in

front of her. Her hands were shaking. She was close to tears.

"Suckers," Gabe said. "They played us for suckers all the way."

"Put them on. Now," Monica said. She smiled. "Unless, of course, you'd care to go inside without them."

45

The suits were like knee-length overcoats of heavy white nylon. Each was equipped with a wide belt, a plastic astronaut's helmet, and a small, flat backpack.

The three of them—Gabe, Kate, and Bernie— slipped the suits on, pulling the helmets over their heads. The helmets were surprisingly lightweight. It was hot inside Gabe's suit. His faceplate had already begun to fog up. Monica came up behind, giving them each a backpack. The backpacks too weighed only a few pounds. Gabe felt sweat trickling down under his arms.

"Cinch those belts up tight," she said. "Mr. Elias wants to keep you all safe and sound. We're just going to put you in a safe place until this all blows over."

Monica backed them against the wall while she stepped into her own suit, zipping it up the front. She flipped a switch on each of their backpacks. The fans inside the packs began to whir. Gabe felt the cool, filtered air blowing into his helmet. His faceplate cleared and he could see again.

"All right." Monica said. "Here we go." She waved them toward the red doors that read NERVE GAS—EXTREME DANGER. The doors opened at their approach, the red lights around the doors blinking a warning.

Monica herded them toward the slowly moving belt. The wide transparent plastic sheets came down the line at a steady pace. The sheets were carried on a succession of soft rubber chains. Tiny vibrating knives between the rubber chains cut the sheets into precise thin strips. The strips, in turn, were pulled off to be cut to length. Gabe was struck by the way the way the whole mechanism operated without human intervention.

"Hey," Bernie said. "Someone's coming." He pointed back down the hallway. They saw a figure moving in the changing room.

"What the hell is this," Monica said.

The red lights began to flash. Someone was coming in through the automatic glass doors.

"Look," Kate said. "It's Sheila."

Sheila came hurrying into the production area in her high heels, making the kind of wig-wagging gesture a person might use to try to stop a passing car. She had evidently put on her helmet in a hurry, for her blond hair was twisted and tangled on top of her head. She carried a cellular phone.

"Please. No," she begged, the sound of her voice thin and tinny through the mask. She stepped up to Monica. "You mustn't do anything to these people," she said. "This is all a horrible mistake."

"This is getting too crazy," Monica said sharply.

She brought the pistol up, leveling it at Sheila's chest. "Where's Elias? He wants to change his plans, he damn well better talk to me directly."

"Yes," Sheila said. "Everything's changed. We're calling the whole thing off. Okay? It's all over."

She looked across at Gabe for the first time. Behind her faceplate Sheila's face was hot and flushed, her makeup running, giving her eyes a bruised look.

"Why? What's happened?" Monica demanded.

"Talk to him," Sheila pleaded, "Please. Here." She dialed in a number and held the phone out to Monica. "Please. Will you please just talk to him for Christ's sake?"

Monica took the phone with her left hand, keeping the gun in her right. She held it up close to her mask, raising her voice to be heard through the faceplate.

"Monica Santini here," she said. "Mr. Elias? What the hell's happening?" She bit her bottom lip and listened.

Gabe exchanged glances with Kate. She closed her eyes and shook her head.

"We have an unexpected visitor down here," Monica said. "Your little blond friend. She says there's been a change of plans." Monica peered through the helmet at Sheila, momentarily turning her back on the others. Gabe watched as Bernie began to back away toward the doors.

"Listen," Monica said. "Things are getting out of control down here. You want me to do that, you'd better come down and help. Wait a minute. Hold it right there." She turned abruptly, leveling her pistol at Bernie.

Bernie had turned and was running toward the door. The phone clattered to the floor. Monica dropped to one knee, supported her right wrist with her left hand, and fired.

The report echoed off the metal walls. There was a sound like a boxer hitting a heavy bag. Monica fired again. The second bullet missed Bernie's head by inches and punctured one of the heavy stainless-steel vats. A stream of liquid shot out under great pressure, filling the air with white vapor.

"Jesus," Kate yelled. "Nerve gas!"

Bernie stumbled and slipped to the floor, writhing and screaming in terror as the steaming liquid sprayed over him. They heard the sound of retching. Bernie was on his knees, his mask off, clutching at his throat.

Monica lowered the gun but remained in her marksman's stance. She reached up with her left hand to make sure her helmet was in place. She was looking across the room, transfixed by what she saw. Her right arm rested on her knee. The pistol was a foot above the floor.

Gabe felt the blood rushing to his face. Bernie had fallen silent now. He had only a few seconds. Gabe shifted his weight forward and kicked the biggest extra point of his life.

Monica fell sideways, swearing, clasping her hand to her chest. The black automatic sailed across the room, coming to rest against the far wall.

Gabe retrieved the gun. It was heavier and colder than he had imagined. Monica looked up at him, holding her hand against her stomach.

Sheila clutched his arm. "Oh, Gabe. I am *so* sorry," she said. "I had no idea he'd go so far. He's crazy, you know. *Really* crazy."

"Wait a minute," Kate said. "Who's this?"

A short, husky figure in a helmet and backpack was coming in the door. They saw that it was Elias.

"Kate? Gabe? What the hell's going on here?" he demanded. "Who was that that just called me?" He glanced down at Bernie. "What's the matter with this man. Good Lord. Has he . . ."

"Ed," Sheila said. "Be careful. There's a nerve gas leak. This . . . this is Monica Santini."

Elias looked Monica up and down, uncomprehending.

Monica looked equally confused. "You're Elias?" she said.

"That's right."

"But who was that other . . ." Monica said. "He told me . . ."

Ed had already stepped past her. He came up to Gabe, reaching out for the pistol. "Put down that gun, Austin," he said. "By God, if this man's been shot, I'm going to hold you personally—"

Something cold and hard slammed into Gabe's left arm. It felt as if he had been hit by a baseball bat. A loud report echoed through the room. He realized that he'd been shot. His whole left side went numb. He felt a warm liquid oozing down under his arm. Surprisingly, there was no pain.

He slipped the gun into his pocket and reached across to draw the upper part of his sleeve together like a tourniquet, trying desperately to seal the hole the bullet had made. His left side was soaked with blood. He was afraid that the bullet might have hit his brachial artery.

Gabe turned to see a tall dark figure in a helmet and backpack.

"My God," Elias said. "It's Storch. Dean, was that you that just shot this man?"

"Shut the fuck up, Ed." Storch smiled strangely, leveling the automatic at Elias. "I've got everything under control."

"The hell you do," Elias said.

"There's a lot you don't know, Ed," Storch said.

"You never really got it, did you? Virazine could have been a billion-dollar drug its first year on the market. But you were just too goddamn stupid to see it."

"Stop being ridiculous," Elias said. "And put that gun down. Jesus, Dean. Let's try to act like halfway civilized people here."

Storch held the pistol against Elias's chest. "Shut up, Ed, for once in your life. I'm in charge right now."

"Damn your impudence," Elias said. "You're finished. I will not stand for this outrageous . . ."

Storch raised the automatic until it pointed directly into Elias's face. "You'll do what you're told, Ed. I have nothing to lose anymore. I swear to God I'll shoot you down like a dog if you try to interfere. Go stand against that wall and shut up." Elias, shaken, backed against the wall.

"You bastard," Sheila hissed. "You didn't tell me you were going to *kill* them."

"I was hoping I wouldn't have to do that, my dear," Storch said. "But extreme conditions require extreme remedies."

Storch stepped across to Gabe, looking at him directly for the first time. There was a real affection and sadness in his eyes.

"I'm sorry about this, old man," he said, his voice full of genuine concern. "This is all turning out very badly. I'm afraid I really had no choice."

46

So what are you planning to do now, Dean? Kill us all?" Gabe felt an icy anger rising inside him. It felt as if his whole body's supply of blood were slowly leaking away.

"I'm sorry, old man." Storch looked down at Bernie's body with an expression of distaste. "You'll have to give me just a moment." He herded the three of them, Gabe, Kate, and Sheila, back against the wall next to Elias. Monica followed behind, still holding her hand.

"So listen, whatever your name is," she said. "I'm getting the hell out of here."

"Stick around," Storch said, waving the barrel of the pistol in her direction. "We'll all go out together."

"Dean . . ." Kate began.

"Stay over there against the wall. All of you," Storch said. "Sheila? Gabe? You come over here."

Storch stood beside the moving assembly line, looking down in fascination at the moving strips of plastic. Gabe and Sheila came forward, standing in front of him. Storch held the gun as if it were a living thing that might turn on him at any moment.

"He's falling apart," Elias said. "Look at him. He's shaking all over."

"Shut up, Ed," Storch said. "I'm sick of hearing your voice. And it would be so easy . . ." He turned to Gabe. "I'm sorry, old man. I'm having a bit of a crisis." His hands were trembling. There was a haunted, desperate look in his eye.

"It seems as if my life has absolutely stopped . . . I don't know what to do. I have no idea . . ." He looked down at the blood dripping from Gabe's hand, appearing to notice Gabe's injury for the first time.

"I say. I'm sorry about that. How's it feeling?" he said.

"It's starting to hurt a little now. What do you say we all get out of here?" Gabe's left arm was flopping like a broken wing at his side. The bleeding had slowed but had not stopped.

"I can't believe I really shot you. I can't believe it. What shall I do, old man? I'm feeling completely lost. I mean it. Will you help me?"

"Sure." Gabe saw that Storch was close to losing control. He glanced back at Kate and Monica. "We all walk out of here," he said. "Slow and easy. Nobody gets hurt."

"I know. I know. God knows, I don't want anyone to be hurt." Storch's voice was as broken and uneven as a child's.

"Sheila? I'm sorry. I'm so, so sorry, my dear. I hope you can forgive me for all this."

"Oh, Dean . . . Of course I will." She reached out and put an arm around him. Gabe let out a long breath as they settled into each other's arms.

Elias took a tentative step toward them. "Yes, let's get everyone out of here safely, if we can," he said. "And I think you owe us all . . . an explanation."

"Yes. Well." Storch shrugged. "I'd arranged for

Kendrick Labs, the big British pharmaceutical firm, to buy Kimberley out. They understood the value of Virazine and would have marketed it aggressively worldwide. It took me a while to convince them that Kimberley would be worth it, since Ed has stifled our research and we didn't have much else in the pipeline. They were going to get rid of Ed and put me on as CEO. Then this company could really have taken off."

Storch looked bitterly at Gabe and shook his head. "You really jinxed that deal for me, old man. As soon as you started turning up those ADRs, everything started going to shit."

Elias stared incredulously at Storch. "You son of a bitch," he said. "So that's why our stock price has been all over the charts. You're finished, Dean. You'll never work in this industry again."

"Not to worry, Ed." Storch smirked. "I've got that little detail all worked out." He stood with one arm around Sheila, as if drawing warmth and comfort. "I'm afraid there's only one way out of this for me now," he said.

"What do you mean?" Sheila looked up at him from under his arm.

Storch took a deep breath. He looked suddenly pleased, as if he had come to an important decision. "Yes," he said. "A little industrial accident." He turned and calmly fired his pistol at each of the two remaining stainless steel vats. Two long plumes of pressurized liquid shot into the room. He then turned his gun on Gabe.

"Monica," he said. "I need you now. Pull their tubes out. All of them."

Before Monica could move, Sheila stepped behind Storch and clawed at his backpack. Storch turned to slap her hands away. Pushing her to the ground, he raised his pistol and calmly shot her in the stomach. The sound was deafening in the enclosed space.

"No!" Gabe hurled himself on Storch's back, clubbing at his head with his one good arm. They went down together. Storch's gun flew across the floor. Storch rolled away and went after it. Somewhere in the distance an alarm went off.

Gabe managed to tug the automatic out of his pocket. He closed one eye, aimed, and squeezed off a shot. It missed Storch's head by inches. Storch jerked backward and ran toward the door.

Gabe turned back to the others. As Monica advanced on Elias, Kate caught her in the stomach with a wicked karate kick. Monica fell hard, the wind knocked out of her. Sheila, moving with great difficulty, crawled toward her. As Gabe watched, she reached across and pulled out Monica's breathing tubes. Monica dropped to her hands and knees, bellowing in pain and terror. The sound of her retching filled the room.

"Come on," Gabe said. "We've got to try to save Sheila."

"Oh, Gabe," Kate said. "Is she . . . ?"

"She's still alive," he said. "We've got to get her out of here. Can you lift her?"

"Yes," Kate said. "I think so. Ed, will you give me a hand?"

Sheila was bleeding heavily but she was still conscious and she still had her helmet on. Monica lay face-down on the floor. She was no longer moving.

"You going to be able to carry her okay?" Gabe asked.

"We're fine," Ed said. "Let's get the hell out of here. You watch out for Storch."

"I'm watching."

Gabe's own bleeding had slowed to a trickle. He

was learning to function without his left arm. They made their way out the glass door. Gabe took the lead, his pistol at the ready, peering down the corridors in every direction. But Storch was nowhere to be seen. They had just reached the doors to the main building by the time the security guards arrived.

47

The ambulance is on its way, Doctor," the young security guard said, standing beside them, white faced, rocking back and forth on his heels, glancing across at Gabe's injured arm. "We'll need to get her out to the front door. They're bringing a stretcher."

Kate sat on the floor, cradling Sheila's head in her lap. Gabe, was applying pressure to the wound in her abdomen, using his one good arm.

"Did you tell them to have an abdominal surgeon standing by?" he asked.

"Yes, sir," the guard said. "They said he'll be there by the time you arrive."

Elias knelt down beside them, his face red with emotion. "Gabe, you make sure that arm gets taken care of," he said. "I'm going upstairs to call the sheriff's office. That bastard Storch. We've got to stop him." He hesitated. "Gabe, Kate," he said at last.

"I just want you to know . . . Well, I'm sorry. For everything."

"He had us all taken in," Gabe said. "Tell Lieutenant Ditmore we're riding in with Sheila. We'll be at the hospital." The older security guard came up the hall, dragging a metal stretcher behind him.

"You guys are going to have to lift her," Gabe said. "I need to keep the pressure on."

He walked along with them, all the way out to the waiting ambulance. The two paramedics transferred Sheila to another stretcher. Gabe stepped up into the van as they loaded her into the ambulance. Kate crowded in beside him. The doors closed behind them and they pulled away.

Sheila's head was tipped back, showing a long white expanse of neck and throat. The ambulance attendant came back and put two fingers up under the angle of her jaw.

"Still hanging in there," he said. "Here, let me get a pressure."

"Don't bother. Just put in the biggest IV you've got," Gabe said. "She's lost a hell of a lot of blood."

The attendant slipped in the IV with an unexpected grace. As they turned off on the Sir Francis Drake exit, Sheila stirred and opened her eyes.

"Kate? Gabe?" Her voice was a faint whisper. Her face was deathly pale. Her hair streamed back over the end of the stretcher. It occurred to Gabe that she already looked like a corpse, yet her pulse was surprisingly strong.

"How . . . how bad is it?" Kate whispered.

"It all depends on what the bullet hit," Gabe said in a low whisper. "If it missed all the vital organs, she could be fine. If it hit a major artery, she may not make it to the hospital."

Gabe tried to calm her fears. "You're going to be

okay, kiddo. We're on our way to the hospital. Hang in there. It won't be long.''

"I'm cold, so cold," Sheila said. "Gabe? Kate? I'm . . . I'm sorry. I was helping him all along. We were going to go away together, after his big deal went through. I was such a fool."

"It's okay," Kate said. "Don't worry now." She crouched beside the stretcher, taking Sheila's hand.

"No. It's *not* okay." Sheila shook her head impatiently, like a woman with no time to waste. "I want . . . want to tell you. He told me . . . Gabe. Wanted me to be lovers with you. Spy on you. Spy on Ed. Tell him everything. I was the one . . . told him you'd written to *60 Minutes*."

Kate looked from Sheila to Gabe with disbelief. Sheila noticed her surprise.

"Kate," she said. "We never . . . did anything. Gabe wouldn't do it. He . . . I think he really loves you. I . . . I got in trouble."

"What did Dean do to you?" Gabe asked.

"He . . . hit me. He made me do bad things. We were going to go away . . . big ranch down in Costa Rica. He was going to paint and I was going to . . ." She began to cough violently. A tiny line of blood trickled down her chin.

"He had it all set up," Sheila said. "Bank accounts. False names. Everything. He was going to . . ." She turned her head to the side and coughed a spattering of blood across the white sheet.

Kate looked questioningly at Gabe. He pressed his lips together and shook his head. They both leaned forward over the pale, frail figure, as if watching the life flow out of her. The attendant slipped a plastic mask over her head and turned on the oxygen. After a few minutes a little color came back into her face. She reached up to push aside the mask.

"I've been doing what he asked . . . so long I couldn't . . . couldn't stop. . . . Do you think . . . Could you ever . . ."

"What?" Kate asked. "Sheila, what?"

"For . . . forgive me? Please . . . please . . ."

Kate looked up at Gabe. Her eyes glistened. She put her arm around Sheila's shoulders.

"Don't think about that now," she said. "You worry about getting yourself well."

Sheila coughed up blood again. When Gabe tried to wipe it away she clutched at his wrist. "You've both been so good to me. Would you . . . just hold me? Just for a minute? Just hold me and don't let me go?"

They held her all the way to the hospital. They were still holding her when the driver pulled into the ambulance entrance of Marin General Hospital.

48

The surgeons repaired Gabe's arm under local anesthetic. He lay on his back on the surgical table, floating in a benzodiazepine daze, his arm bound to a heavy board. He listened as the vascular surgeons discussed what they should do to repair his torn vessels. From time to time they would ask him to move his fingers this way or that.

The whole business with his arm was like a tiny candle flame at the far end of a long, dark tunnel. Gabe felt as if he were swimming in a comforting sea of warm, thick liquid honey. The familiar voices had come to comfort him. They seemed to hover just above the bank of surgical lights, asking themselves if perhaps he was about to join them. *Not yet,* they decided. *No, not yet.*

The surgeons put his arm in a sling and made him sit in a wheelchair. Young men in green scrubs kept asking him to count backward by sevens. A nurse brought him a glass of water with a plastic straw. Then they all hurried away to care for other patients.

After what seemed a long time an orderly wheeled Gabe to a waiting room where Kate was talking to a beefy young man in a Marin County sheriff's jacket. She stood up quickly and burst into tears.

"Oh, God, Gabe. I'm so glad you're okay. They kept you in there so *long.*" She wiped her eyes with a tissue and crossed the room to hug him.

Gabe found this all mildly confusing. Kate was beautiful and vulnerable in her happiness and her grief. It felt as though he were trying to get his mind to go through a particular door. But the door was closed and there was no key. There was not even a keyhole.

"Dr. Bradley says the surgery went fine," she said. "There'll be no permanent damage. But you're going to be pretty sore for a while. Oh. This is Hank Peavy. From the sheriff's office."

Peavy was an earnest, clean-shaven young man with a thick red neck and spots of color in his cheeks. He held his trooper's hat on his lap.

"How's Sheila?" Gabe asked. The words seemed to come up from some closed chamber deep inside him. It was as if a radio speaker had been implanted in his chest.

Kate smiled. "They said it was remarkable that the bullet didn't hit any major organs," she said. "She was out of the operating room before you were. They just moved her upstairs. Room 417. She's going to be okay."

"How about Storch?"

"We checked the local airports," the deputy said. "Dr. Storch has a reservation on an afternoon plane to Costa Rica. They're going to pick him up when he tries to board the plane."

Gabe shook his head. "That doesn't figure," he said. "This is a very smart guy. I really can't believe . . ."

The deputy regarded Gabe with a polite disdain. "I wouldn't know about that, sir," he said. "The sheriff himself is headed down to pick him up."

A loud, clanging bell went off in the hall. The alarm echoed in Gabe's ears like a prophetic warning. The deputy jumped to his feet and hurried to the door.

"What the hell's that?" he said.

An orderly in a green scrub suit trotted into the room. "We've got some smoke in a downstairs hallway, officer. We need to evacuate all the patients from the first floor. We could use your help. You too, ma'am."

"You guys go ahead," Gabe said. He set the brakes on his wheelchair and pushed himself to a standing position. His arm hurt, but his balance was good and he could still walk. "I can get myself out. Kate, you want to give me the keys? I'll wait for you in the car."

"Gabe, are you sure?"

He nodded. "I'll take it real easy," he said.

He made his way down the hallway and took the

walk out to the parking lot a step at a time. It was a cool, sunny California day. Joggers were passing by on the trail across the street. A light breeze rustled the leaves of the trees. There were birds darting and singing overhead and planter boxes with bright flowers.

It seemed to Gabe that time had slowed and the pressure was finally off. It was very pleasant to be here. He found that walking took all his attention. He was so preoccupied by the flowers and the bright blue sky that he nearly walked past the green Jaguar.

He retraced his steps and walked around the sleek sedan. It was Storch's car, sure enough. The yellow and green golf cap lay in a corner of the back seat.

He leaned against the car, listening to the echoing fire alarm. It occurred to him that Storch must have set it off to lure the hospital staffers away from Sheila's room. A motherly woman with short salt-and-pepper hair was pushing a frail hairless man in a wheelchair along the row of cars where Gabe was standing.

"Good afternoon," she said.

"Good afternoon."

She looked him over in a frank, benign appraisal. "Are you locked out?" she asked.

"No," Gabe said. "No. Just thinking."

This seemed to cheer her considerably. She nodded her approval. "Well, good enough," she said. "You have a good day then." She pushed her silent husband on through the dappled shade.

Gabe repositioned his arm in his sling, pushed himself away from the car, and headed slowly back across the parking lot toward the hospital.

49

Gabe came staggering up out of the echoing stairwell, the pain in his arm pulsing with each heartbeat. He had begun to hear the voices again.

The nurses' station on the fourth floor was deserted. The alarm bell at the far end of the empty corridor continued to ring. The door to 417 stood open. Gabe could see only a long green curtain inside.

He crossed the hallway and stepped quietly into the room. The hospital bed had been rolled into a far corner. Sheila lay there, unmoving, a clear bag of IV fluid dripping slowly into her arm. A surgical drain hung from her bandaged abdomen. Dean Storch was standing at the foot of her bed. He was holding a large syringe. The voices were loud in Gabe's ears.

Storch was intent on his work and had not seen him. Gabe saw that he was having trouble with the tourniquet. Storch put down the needle and began rewrapping it, using both hands. Gabe stepped up behind him and picked up the syringe.

"What are you trying to do, Dean? Finish the job?" he said. His voice was loud in his ears.

Storch jerked back from the bed. The tourniquet slipped off Sheila's arm and fell to the floor. He took a step away from the bedside, hands raised to his shoulders, palms forward, shaking his head.

"Jesus, Gabe. You just don't quit, do you?" Storch tried to force a laugh but broke into a hacking cough instead. He was wearing a crisp gray suit and a fresh white shirt. He looked haunted and exhausted. His face was terribly pale.

Gabe looked down at the syringe. "What's this you're giving her?" he asked.

"Just a little Demerol to help calm her down and keep her comfortable for the trip."

Demerol is a powerful narcotic pain reliever. "Really?" Gabe said. "How much?"

"I believe it was three hundred milligrams." Gabe heard a note of uncertainty in Storch's voice. As much as Storch might know about theoretical pharmacology, his total lack of clinical experience would have to make him uneasy.

"Big mistake," Gabe said. "The way Demerol interacts with MAO inhibitors, and the Virazine she took at your crazy press conference, she could go straight into a coma, or worse."

"What do you mean?" Storch looked down at the syringe. "Demerol can't trigger hypertensive crisis, can it?"

"No, but the interaction's often lethal, nonetheless. But you must know that, Dean. I don't think you want to take her anywhere."

"You've got it all wrong, old man. Sheila . . . well . . . she's the dearest thing in the world to me."

"Sure. That's why you shot her."

"I feel terrible about that. Terrible. I only hope I can make it . . ."

"Yeah, right. Just like you must feel terrible about trying to kill Gertrude. I bet she called you that morning, all excited with what she'd found."

Storch looked down at the floor. "Actually, I knew about the reaction long before that."

"Sure. Your friend Howard must have told you all about it."

Storch shook his head and turned away. "That was very difficult. Howard and I went way back. He just wouldn't listen to reason."

Gabe looked at the sleeping figure in the hospital bed. "You were really planning to take her with you?"

"She's all I have, old man." Storch said. A wry smile played across his face. "She's been the only constant thing in my life. Costa Rica will be different. We're going to start a whole new . . ."

"Don't talk crazy," Gabe said. "You'll never get out of here, Dean. They're watching the airports. Listen—I'm going to phone down and set it up for you to surrender to the sheriff's deputy downstairs." He picked up the bedside phone. "It'll go a lot—" Gabe frowned. The phone was dead. He saw that the cord had been pulled out of the wall.

Storch smiled. "I'm afraid not, old man." He took out a white handkerchief and pressed it to his lips. "Brian?" he said. "You want to come do the honors here?"

Ray Brody's nurse-bodyguard stepped out from behind the green curtain, an uneasy smile on his face. The shiny revolver looked small in his massive hand.

"Hello there, Doc," he said.

"I doubt he's armed, but you better check him out," Storch said.

Brian nodded and stepped forward. "Let me take that off your hands, Doc," he said, taking the hypodermic and replacing it carefully on the bedside table. "You want to turn around for me? Hands against the wall?"

Gabe turned around. "I can't move my left arm," he said.

"Hey. No problem. No problem at all." He began to pat Gabe down, none too gently.

"Okay, Doc," Brian said. "You can relax now." He turned to Storch. "Clean as a whistle."

Gabe turned around to find himself looking into the dark eye of the revolver. The voices whispered comfortingly into his ear. The back of his neck was suddenly cold with sweat. He took a step toward the bed, looking down at the motionless form under the sheet.

"I can't figure her out," Gabe said. "She seems so devoted to you. What have you got on her, anyway?"

Storch looked up quickly. He looked mildly embarrassed. "I'm afraid you have it all wrong, old man," he said. "Sheila is my sister."

"Your *sister?*"

Storch nodded, a pained smile on his face. "Brian, if you please, I'd like you to tape his wrists to the railing of the bed. I'll just give him a little injection to keep him relaxed until we get to where we have to go." To Gabe he said, "Yes, why not? It's our dirty little secret. I'm sure she must have told you her Little Orphan Annie story?"

"I guess I missed that one."

"We were very close as children. When we were teenagers we were put out for adoption to different homes. Years later, she hired a detective to track me down. I was at Oxford at the time. She helped me out of a real jam. We had different names, separate identities. I decided to keep it that way. We kept up the appearance of a superficial relationship. I was able to pass her off as my protégée. And, eventually, as my subordinate."

Gabe shook his head. "You're sicker than I thought," he said.

Storch smiled, remembering. "She was a wonderful weapon in the corporate wars, old man. The men fell before her like dominoes, Ed and most of the top Kimberley execs among them. You were one of her few failures. As long as the man resisted, she would pursue him with an obsessive intensity. But once she'd had her victory, she lost all interest. I'm afraid she found the actual act rather repugnant."

"Dr. Storch," Brian said. "I hate to interrupt. But we haven't got forever."

"All right, Brian," Storch said. "Let's get him taped up."

Gabe felt the bodyguard's hand on his shoulder. "No time for that, boss," Brian said. "Let me do this my way."

Gabe saw the gun coming toward his head. He tried to pull away, but the blow caught him high on the cheekbone.

It felt as if a bomb had exploded in his skull. His mouth began to fill with blood. He felt the side of his head puffing up, even as his legs went out from under him. A moment later he was lying on the floor under the curtain, coming up slowly out of a blank darkness.

"Really, Brian," he heard Storch say. "That was hardly necessary."

"You can inject him with anything you want now, Doc. He'll be out for a good ten, fifteen minutes. You're going to want to ice the guy anyway, right?"

"Shut up, Brian. You talk too goddamn much."

"All right, all right. I'm sorry. So let's get your girlfriend disconnected and you shoot him up with whatever and we'll split."

The pain in his head nearly overwhelmed Gabe's

ability to think. The voices fluttered about him. *In extremity,* one of his teachers had liked to say, *endorphins help get us through.* It occurred to him that endorphins might be the biochemical basis of angels. He wondered, vaguely, if he might have a concussion.

When he was finally able to open his eyes, Gabe saw that he was screened from their view by the green curtain. He got a hand on the windowsill and with great difficulty pulled himself to his feet. Staying behind the curtain, he moved up behind the two men working over the bed.

The syringe of Demerol still lay on the bedside table. He waited until Brian lifted Sheila into his arms, then reached out from behind the curtain and picked it up. Neither Storch nor Brian seemed to notice.

Sheila lay limply in the Brian's arms. Storch was removing her IV. Gabe felt the powerful thrill of cold anger rising inside him. His head and his left arm burned with pain. But his breathing was regular and the syringe felt comfortingly familiar in his hand.

Storch was leaning forward, tucking the blanket around Sheila, when Gabe stepped out from behind the curtain and came up behind him.

"Dr. Storch," Brian said, looking up. "Look out."

In one smooth motion, Gabe drove the needle through Storch's trousers, deep into his right buttock. He pressed the plunger, injecting the full contents of the syringe into the muscle. He felt like a Stone Age man, driving his spear into a game animal after a long hunt.

Storch bellowed. He reached back incredulously, grasping at the empty syringe still dangling from his flesh. He pulled it out of his buttock and threw it across the room.

"What the hell!" he wailed. "Gabe. You son of a bitch . . ."

"A little present, Dean," Gabe said. "Now you'll know how Lindsey and the others felt. You've got the drug—from the press conference. You've got the trigger—three hundred milligrams of Demerol. And with all your trips to Japan, you must have had a flu shot. You're dead meat, buddy. It's just a matter of time. Unless you come down to the emergency room and let me get you some Thorazine."

He saw the panic rising in Storch's face. Brian dropped Sheila roughly back onto the bed. She let out a little cry but did not open her eyes.

"All right, Doc," Brian said, advancing slowly toward him. "You're going to shut up and be a good boy now."

"It's lights-out time, baby," Gabe said to Storch. "Demerol is one of the most powerful MAO inhibitor triggers there is. You've got two choices. You can ignore it and try to run. If you do, you'll die a painful, horrible death. Sweating. Fever. Seizures. A horrible headache. Coma. Then you stop breathing."

Storch looked at Gabe with cold hatred. "I've changed my mind about your injection, old man," he said. "I had been *thinking* of a nice little sedative. But after this latest little trick, I think I'll make that a double dose of potassium."

"Come on down with me right now," Gabe said. "I can start treating you before the reaction comes on."

"Jesus, Dr. Storch," Brian said. "You don't look so good. You sure you're feeling okay?"

"Get him, Brian," Storch said. "I'm not about to listen to any more of this bullshit."

Brian came up from behind and got an arm around Gabe's waist, immobilizing him.

"You're going to be developing a horrible headache any minute now," Gabe said. "It might take five minutes or fifteen . . ."

"He's bluffing," Storch said. "It's nothing but a desperate attempt to fuck with my mind."

"Brian, you try to get him out of here without treatment you're going to be driving a dead man," Gabe said.

"I want him on his knees," Storch said. "His ankles tied back under the bed, with both his arms extended out along the rails. One good injection deserves another, don't you think?"

Brian positioned Gabe's arms until he was spread-eagled on the rail of Sheila's hospital bed. Brian wound the tape around and around until Gabe could barely move. His left arm burned with pain.

Brian stepped back, checking his work with satisfaction. "There you go, Dr. Storch. That should hold him."

"How does it feel, Dean?" Gabe felt clear and strong and fearless.

"Feeling just fine, old man. Best I've felt in months."

Sheila's voice came from behind Gabe's back. "Dean? Is that you?"

Storch hurried to the other side of the bed. "It's me, darling. How are you feeling?"

"Awful. My stomach hurts." She pushed a button on her remote control and the head of the bed moved slowly upward. "What are Gabe and Brian doing here?" she asked.

"You're in the hospital, darling. I've come back to get you. Like I promised. Brian is going to carry you to the car."

Gabe looked back over his shoulder at the two of them. He couldn't help but notice an unmistakable family resemblance, the angular pale faces, the wide eyes, the nervous, hungry look, the skin close to the bone. He marveled that he had never seen it before.

"Oh, Gabe," she said. "They've got you all tied up. I'm sorry. It's all my fault." Sheila reached out a hand to touch his arm. "Did Dean tell you he was my brother?"

"He told me," Gabe said. "That explains a lot."

She shook her head, smiling a ghastly smile. "Don't ever let him tell you he doesn't care about his family. Did he tell you he was the one who was slipping his hand into my underpants for all those years?" she said. "How old was I in the beginning, Dean? Seven? Eight?"

"And how old was I?" Storch said, his face coloring. "Nine or ten? You were not exactly unwilling."

"Now he's all embarrassed," Sheila said. "I'm sorry, brother. I'll be a good girl. I'll keep my mouth shut. I'll fuck anybody you ask me to. I won't tell anyone anything, ever again. I'll be good. I promise."

Storch had taken a smaller vial and needle from his bag. He wrapped the rubber tourniquet around Gabe's right bicep, peered down at the veins on the inside of his elbow, and picked up the syringe.

"So what are you going to do to him, brother?" Sheila said. "Why is he all tied up like that?"

"I'm just giving him a shot to make him sleep, darling. We want to make sure he doesn't spoil our plans. Any last words, Gabe? For old times' sake?"

Gabe felt his heart beating. He pulled and struggled with all his strength, but his arms were well secured and the tape did not budge.

"Last chance, Dean," Gabe said. "The MAO inhibitor reaction isn't going to be pretty. I think they'd go easy on you. It's not like you'd be some big threat to society now.''

"Let's see if I still remember how to do this," Storch said. Gabe watched in fascination as Storch palpated a large vein. He felt the sharp needle tip touch his skin.

"Okay, Brian," Storch said. "You get Sheila and I'll . . .''

The dark tip of the needle hovered above Gabe's arm. Storch stepped back and stood with his feet apart, putting the needle down on the bedside table and bringing his hands to his temples. "Oh, my God," he said. "My head." His knees buckled and he dropped to the floor.

"Dr. Storch?" Brian said.

"He's not going anywhere, Brian," Gabe said. He felt his heart beating like a jackhammer in his chest. "If you want to save him, and yourself, cut me lose so I can treat him. Then you can get the hell out of here.''

"Oh, God, it's awful. Awful." Storch said. He tried to push himself up to his hands and knees, but his arms slipped out from beneath him. "Oh, my God. Gabe," he begged. "Help me.''

"Dr. Storch?" Brian said.

"He's too far gone, Brian," Gabe said. "He can't even hear you. He'll be dead in minutes unless you . . .''

Brian's eyes shifted back and forth between Gabe and the figure on the floor. Gabe knew by the look on his face that he was beginning to lose control.

"I . . . I really never wanted anyone to get hurt," Brian said. He took out his pocket knife and began to cut through Gabe's bonds. "Sorry about your face, Doc. You're going to have a hell of a black eye.''

By the time Gabe was loose, Storch was unconscious. He lay on his side on the floor like a child, defenseless and vulnerable.

"Gabe?" Sheila said. "Is he dying?"

"Yes. I think so." The pain in Gabe's face was much worse when he knelt. He stood up suddenly, putting out his good arm to steady himself. Sheila began to cry, and Gabe began to hear the voices again.

The fire alarm came to an abrupt stop. Gabe leaned against the wall in the sudden silence of the deserted hospital. He had only to walk away, and it would all be over.

Storch had begun to shake with a seizure. He could stop breathing at any second.

Sheila was looking down over the bed rail, her eyes puffy and red. "What . . . what are you going to do?"

Gabe shrugged. He thought of Lindsey and the others. Then he walked slowly toward the door. He stumbled out to the deserted nurses' station, picked up the phone, and dialed the emergency room.

The whole ER crew was on the floor in less than three minutes. With a crash cart, an ambu bag, and a large dose of Thorazine.

50

It was 7:55 on Monday morning. Gabe was standing at the counter in the back of the radio room at St. Catherine's emergency department, his left arm in a sling, finishing up his charts. He was concentrating so hard that he did not hear Kate's soft knock at the door.

"Well. You look right at home," she said, crossing the room to kiss him. "Have a good weekend?" She was wearing jeans and a black turtleneck under a gray tweed jacket. Her round Irish face was fresh from sleep, her hair still damp from the shower.

He leaned back against the counter, resting his weight on his good elbow. "It was jumping last night. But it quieted down about two this morning. I must have gotten three or four hours of sleep."

"Your face looks a lot better today." She twisted her lower jaw to one side, raising her eyebrows. "I can't believe you wanted to come to work after all . . ."

He shrugged. She would probably never understand his attraction to the ER, the small, bright cubicles with their waxed tile floors reflecting scene after scene of intense human experience. Well, he decided, that was all right too.

"I was tempted to beg off," he said. "But once they finally put me back on the schedule . . ."

"Yeah. I know," she said. "You just couldn't resist. So the drug charges were dropped?"

He nodded. "The board decided that in light of my upstanding character, someone must have planted the stuff in my locker. What happened at the press conference? I was too busy last night to turn it on."

"About what we expected," she said. "Ed took Virazine off the market. He said some very nice things about you and me. Storch was faking the data, hiding the ADRs.

"When he realized the buyout was dead in the water he bought a million dollars' worth of puts through a dozen different brokers. He figured that when the Virazine story broke, Kimberley's stock would plummet, and he'd make millions overnight. He'd arranged to have the money wired to a numbered account in the Cayman Islands. It would have been no sweat getting it from Costa Rica."

"So how far down did the stock go?"

"From one-forty to seventy-nine." Kate made a face. "He must have sixty million sitting in that bank account. Where he can't touch it. The courts will have a great time trying to sort that one out."

"Pretty slick."

"Stu Zolar was there. You're back on the KSF payroll, beginning today. They're getting great mileage out of you already. All that footage from the press conference is being rebroadcast all over the country as a KSF–copyrighted story. And you'll love this—there was a crew there from *60 Minutes*. They want to do a piece on Monica's impersonation."

"Did you check their credentials?"

She shook her head. "I should have. Oh, did you

see this? I didn't realize he'd had such a serious stroke."

She passed Gabe the morning edition of the *Chronicle*. A large story at the bottom of the front page showed a photograph of Storch in a flimsy hospital gown, sitting in a wheelchair. One side of his face was paralyzed. The headline read FORMER KIMBERLEY EXEC FACES MURDER CHARGE.

"Ed says there's going to be a civil suit," Kate said. "He expects the jury to give every penny Storch owns to the victims' families. Sheila checked herself into a drug rehab program. She's determined to make a clean break. And Gertrude's out of her coma. She's going to be okay."

Gabe nodded. "Lew Watkins called me last night."

"So it looks like we've only got one problem left to deal with," Kate said.

"Yeah? What's that?"

"Getting you out of the hospital," she said. "I'm starving."

"I'm out of here." He said, dropping his completed paperwork in the basket. "Let's go, before they find something else for me to do."

Gabe checked out at the desk and followed Kate through the sliding glass doors of the ambulance entrance.

They left the hospital arm in arm, in search of their long-postponed breakfast. Gabe saw that Kate was looking up at him strangely.

"What's the matter?" he said.

"I just want to ask you one thing," she said. "Did you ever think about just letting him die?"

He nodded. "I guess I came pretty close."

"What stopped you?"

"I was standing there thinking about it," he said. "My face and arm were hurting like hell. I was ready to walk away. Then all of a sudden I'm back at our med school graduation. You remember that?"

She shook her head. "I didn't wait around for graduation."

"It was a long time ago, but I still remember," he said. "We all marched in wearing our blue robes and our funny hats. We stood there in the sun with our hands on our hearts. We vowed that we would first do no harm. We would abstain from all manner of mischief and corruption. And we promised—for whatever it was worth—that we would prescribe no deadly drug."